Midwifery Essentials

Antenatal

For Elsevier:

Commissioning Editor: Mairi McCubbin
Development Editor: Sheila Black
Project Manager: Christine Johnston
Designer: Charlotte Murray, Kirsteen Wright
Illustrations Manager: Merlyn Harvey

Midwifery Essentials

Volume 2 **Antenatal**

Helen Baston BA(Hons) MMedSci PhD ADM PGDipEd RN RM

Lead Midwife for Education; Supervisor of Midwives, Mother & Infant Research Unit, Department of Health Sciences, University of York, York, UK

Jennifer Hall MSc ADM PGDip(HE) RN RM

Senior Lecturer in Midwifery, Faculty of Health and Life Sciences, University of the West of England, Bristol, UK

Foreword by

Deirdre Daly BSc(Hons) MSc(Health Care Ethics & Law) MSc(Midwifery) PGCertAdultEd DipMidwifery RGN RM

Lecturer in Midwifery, University of Dublin Trinity College, Dublin, Republic of Ireland; President, European Midwives Association 2005–2009

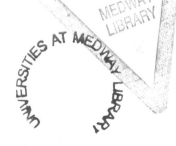

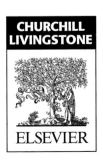

CHURCHILL
LIVINGSTONE

ELSEVIER

Edinburgh London New York Oxford Philadelphia St Louis Sydney Toronto 2009

CHURCHILL LIVINGSTONE
ELSEVIER

© 2009 Elsevier Limited. All rights reserved.

First published 2009
   Reprinted 2009, 2010

ISBN 978-0-443-10354-4

British Library Cataloguing in Publication Data
A catalogue record for this book is available from the British Library

Library of Congress Cataloging in Publication Data
A catalog record for this book is available from the Library of Congress

Notice

Knowledge and best practice in this field are constantly changing. As new research and experience broaden our knowledge, changes in practice, treatment and drug therapy may become necessary or appropriate. Readers are advised to check the most current information provided (i) on procedures featured or (ii) by the manufacturer of each product to be administered, to verify the recommended dose or formula, the method and duration of administration, and contraindications. It is the responsibility of the practitioner, relying on their own experience and knowledge of the patient, to make diagnoses, to determine dosages and the best treatment for each individual patient, and to take all appropriate safety precautions. To the fullest extent of the law, neither the Publisher nor the Editors assumes any liability for any injury and/or damage to persons or property arising out or related to any use of the material contained in this book.

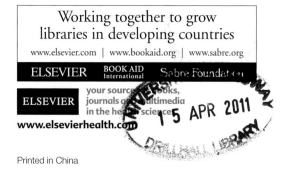

Working together to grow libraries in developing countries

www.elsevier.com | www.bookaid.org | www.sabre.org

ELSEVIER   BOOK AID International   Sabre Foundation

ELSEVIER
your source for books, journals and multimedia in the health sciences
www.elsevierhealth.com

1 5 APR 2011

Printed in China

Contents

I believe that the foundations for a good birth and good parenting are laid down in the antenatal period. For many women, antenatal care is their first introduction to any formal healthcare service and there is no doubt that a positive experience in the antenatal period can empower women. A positive experience for women requires a midwife who is informed and willing to engage with women in an open, transparent and moral manner from the first meeting through to birth and beyond. This in turn requires a thorough knowledge of the very basics and essentials of antenatal care.

Jennifer Hall and Mel Baston have written a text that gives all midwives and midwifery students the essentials to becoming such a midwife. The essentials of antenatal care and the content of the antenatal visits are presented in this easy-to-read, accessible text. The use of vignettes, case examples and links to reflective points, research, evidence and policy make the process real and easily transferable into practice.

As a practising midwife and Lecturer in Midwifery, I can readily see how this text will benefit the women for whom I provide care and the midwifery students I help inform.

As the President of the European Midwives Association and in the context of the free movement of midwives, EU enlargement and discussions on the existence of a 'European midwife', I believe this text offers a wonderful introduction to the models and content of antenatal care and that it is an essential text for all newly appointed midwives in the UK. While the models of care described are applicable to some or all parts of England, Scotland, Wales and Northern Ireland, much of the content is applicable to those of us practising in the Republic of Ireland and to midwifery colleagues in Europe. I would go so far as to suggest that a text such as this, describing and outlining the options for and essential content of antenatal care (and labour, birth and the postnatal period) would be advantageous for all countries.

While pregnant women's wants and needs may differ according to each individual, all pregnant women need safe, competent care from a safe, competent, knowledgeable midwife – a midwife who knows the basics and essentials of care and can build on this to meet the needs of each individual woman in their care.

If you get antenatal care right, everything else can follow easily, safely and positively for women. If you get the basics of antenatal care wrong, or inadvertently miss the essentials of care, you risk irredeemably jeopardizing the woman, her labour and birth, and her family.

Dublin, 2009   Deirdre Daly

To contribute to the provision of sensitive, safe and effective maternity care for women and their families is a privilege. Childbirth is a life-changing event for women. Those around them and those who input into any aspect of pregnancy, labour, birth or the postnatal period can positively influence how this event is experienced and perceived. In order to achieve this, maternity carers continually need to reflect on the services they provide and strive to keep up-to-date with developments in clinical practice. They should endeavour to ensure that women are central to the decisions made and that real choices are offered and supported by skilled practitioners.

This book is the second volume in a series of texts based on the popular 'Midwifery Basics' series published in *The Practising Midwife* journal. Since their publication, there have been many requests from students, midwives and supervisors to combine the articles into a handy text to provide a resource for learning and refreshment of midwifery knowledge and skills. The books have remained true to the original style of the articles and have been updated and expanded to create a user-friendly source of information. They are also intended to stimulate debate and require the reader both to reflect on their current practice, local policies

and procedures and to challenge care that is not woman-centred. The use of scenarios enables the practitioner to understand the context of maternity care and explore their role in its safe and effective provision.

There are many dimensions to the provision of woman-centred care that practitioners need to consider and understand. To aid this process, a jigsaw model has been introduced, with the aim of encouraging the reader to explore maternity care from a wide range of perspectives. For example, how does a midwife obtain consent from a woman for a procedure, maintain a safe environment during the delivery of care and make the most of the opportunity to promote health? What are the professional and legal issues in relation to the procedure and is this practice based on the best available evidence? Which members of the multi-professional team contribute to this aspect of care and how is it influenced by the way care is organized? Each aspect of the jigsaw should be considered during the assessment, planning, implementation and evaluation of woman-centred maternity care.

Midwifery Essentials: Antenatal is about the provision of safe and effective antenatal care. It comprises 10 chapters, each written to stand alone or be read in succession. The introductory chapter sets the scene, exploring the role of the midwife in the context of professional and national guidance. The jigsaw model for midwifery care is introduced and explained, providing a framework to explore each aspect of antenatal care provision, described in subsequent chapters. Chapter 2 explores the options available for women. It outlines the models of care and the range of professionals who may contribute to it. Chapter 3 describes the booking history and how the midwife can involve the woman in decisions about her care. Chapters 4 and 5 explore how maternal health can be optimized and monitored throughout pregnancy and Chapter 6 focuses specifically on women's emotional wellbeing during pregnancy. Chapters 7 and 8 examine the various blood tests that may be offered to women and how antenatal screening for fetal abnormality is approached. Chapter 9 explores how the wellbeing of the growing fetus is monitored during pregnancy. This volume concludes with Chapter 10, which discusses how women can prepare for the birth and how the midwife facilitates this process. This book therefore prepares the reader to provide safe, evidence-based, woman-centred maternity care. Subsequent books in the series explore contemporary intrapartum and postnatal care for women and their families, exploring the role of the midwife as a member of the multi-professional team.

Helen Baston

York and Bristol, 2009   Jennifer Hall

Acknowledgements

In the process of writing there are always people behind the scenes who support or add to the development of the book. We would specifically like to thank Mary Seager, formerly Senior Commissioning Editor at Elsevier, for her initial vision, support and prompting to turn the journal articles from *The Practising Midwife* into a readable volume. In addition, none of us could have completed this project without the love, support, patience and endless cups of tea and coffee provided by our partners and children. To you we owe our greatest gratitude.

Chapter 1

Introduction

This book is the second in the *Midwifery Essentials* series aimed at student midwives and those who support them in clinical practice. It focuses on antenatal care for low-risk women beginning with how antenatal care is organized and then taking the reader through the pregnancy journey. Scenarios are used throughout the book to facilitate learning and assist the reader to apply this knowledge to their own practice areas. In particular, one woman, Joanna, is followed throughout the course of her pregnancy, to illustrate how different issues become more pertinent or prominent at different times along the way. The mantra for contemporary maternity care is choice, access and continuity of care within a safe and effective service (Department of Health 2004; Department of Health 2007). The focus of this book is to explore ways in which this aspiration can become a reality for women and their families.

The aim of this introductory chapter is:

- To introduce the 'jigsaw model' for exploring effective midwifery practice.

The jigsaw model (Fig. 1.1) is used throughout the book, except for Chapter 2, which provides a general introduction to the various models of antenatal care currently available.

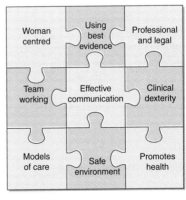

Fig. 1.1 Jigsaw model: dimensions of effective midwifery care

Midwifery care model

One of the purposes of this series is to consider the care of women and their babies from an holistic viewpoint. This means considering the care from a physical, emotional, psychological, spiritual, social and cultural context. To do this we have devised a jigsaw model of care that will encourage the reader to consider individual aspects of care, while recognizing that these aspects go to make up part of the whole person being cared for.

This model will be used to reflect on the clinical scenarios described in the chapters. It shows the dimensions for effective maternity care and each should be considered during the assessment, planning, implementation and evaluation of an aspect of care.

The pieces of the jigsaw (Fig. 1.1) clearly interlink with each other and each is needed for the provision of safe, holistic care. When one is missing the picture will be incomplete and care will not reach its potential. Each aspect of the model is described below in more detail. It is recommended that when an aspect of midwifery care is being evaluated each piece of the jigsaw is addressed. Consider the questions pertaining to each piece of the jigsaw and work through those that are relevant to the clinical situation you face.

Woman-centred care

The provision of woman-centred care was one of the central messages of the policy document *Changing Childbirth*

(Department of Health 1993) which turned the focus of maternity care from meeting the needs of the professionals to listening and responding to the aspirations of women. This is further enforced in the *National service framework* (Department of Health 2004) and *Maternity matters* (Department of Health 2007) and is an expectation of midwifery practice (NMC 2004) and pre-registration education (NMC 2009). When considering particular aspects of care the questions that need to be addressed to ensure that the woman's care is woman-centred include:

- Was the woman involved in the development of her care plan and its subsequent implementation?
- Should her family or carers also be involved?
- How can I ensure that she remains involved in further decisions about her care?
- What are the implications of undertaking or not undertaking this procedure on this particular woman or baby?
- Are there any factors that I need to consider that might influence the results of this procedure for this woman and their impact on her?
- How does this procedure fit in with the woman's hopes, expectations and meanings?
- Is now the most appropriate time to undertake this procedure?

Using best evidence

The NMC Code states 'you must deliver care based on the best available evidence or best practice' (NMC 2008:04). Midwifery evidence includes many aspects (Wickham 2004) and the decisions a midwife makes about her practice will be influenced by a range of factors. However, in the statement above, care should be based as much as possible on the 'best' evidence, and reflect national guidance (NICE 2008) as appropriate.

Questions that need to be addressed when exploring the evidence base of care include:

- What is already known about this aspect of care?
- What is the justification for the choices made about care?
- What is the research evidence available on this procedure/test?
- Do local guidelines reflect best evidence?
- Was a midwife involved in development of local/national guidelines?
- Who represents users of maternity services on groups where guidelines are developed?
- What midwifery research project has your Trust been involved in?
- Where do you go first in order to identify sources of best evidence?

Professional and legal

Midwives who practise in the United Kingdom must adhere to the rules and guidance of the Nursing and Midwifery Council (NMC). The Code states:

As a professional you are accountable for actions and omissions in your practice and must always justify your decisions. You must always act lawfully, whether those laws relate to your professional practice or personal life.

(NMC 2008:01)

Midwives are therefore required to comply with English law and the rules and regulations of their employers.

Questions that need to be addressed to ensure that the woman's care fulfils statutory obligations include:

- Is this procedure expected to be an integral part of education prior to qualification?
- How do the midwives rules relate to this care/test?
- Which NMC proficiencies relate to this care/test?
- How does the NMC Code relate to this care/test?
- Is there any other NMC guidance applicable to this care/test?
- Are there any national or international guidelines for this care/test?
- Are there any legal issues underpinning the use of this care/ test?

Team working

Midwives work as part of a team of professionals who each bring particular skills and perspectives to the care of women and their families. The NMC Code requires registrants to 'keep colleagues informed when you are sharing care with others' and 'work with colleagues to monitor the quality of your work and maintain the safety of those in your care' (NMC 2008:03). It also states:

- You must work cooperatively within teams and respect the skills, expertise and contributions of your colleagues
- You must be willing to share your skills and experience for the benefit of your colleagues
- You must consult and take advice from colleagues when appropriate
- You must treat your colleagues fairly and without discrimination (NMC 2008:03).

Midwives rules and standards also requires midwives to refer any woman or baby whose condition deviates from normal to an appropriate health professional (NMC 2004:16).

Questions that need to be addressed to ensure that the woman's care makes appropriate use of the multi-professional team include:

- Does this test fall within my role?
- Have I acknowledged the limitations of my professional knowledge?
- Who else will need to be involved to interpret the results?
- Where should these results be recorded for all to see?
- Who will I involve if the results are outside normal parameters?
- How can I facilitate effective team working with this woman?
- Will another person be required to assist with this care?
- When will they be available and how can I access them?

Effective communication

Central to any interaction between a woman and the midwife is effective communication. It is essential that the midwife is aware of the cues she is giving to the woman during the care she provides. Time is often pressured in midwifery, both in the community and hospital setting, but it is important to convey to the woman that she is the focus of your attention. Taking time to explain what you are going to do, and why, is crucial if she is going to trust that you are acting in her best interest. Questions that need to be addressed to ensure that effective communication is achieved before, during and after any aspect of antenatal care include:

- What information needs to be given in order for the woman to choose whether this is the right decision for her?
- Has she given consent?
- Is she clear what the care/test entails?
- In what ways could the information be given?
- What should be said during the care/test?
- What should be observed in the woman's behaviour during the care/test?
- What should be communicated to the woman after the care/test?
- How and where should recording of the care/test and its results be made?

Clinical dexterity

Midwifery is a profession that requires the practitioner to have a range of knowledge and a repertoire of clinical skills. The midwife continues to learn new skills throughout her working life and is accountable for maintaining and developing her practice as new ways of working are introduced (NMC 2008:04).

Questions that need to be addressed to ensure that the woman's care is provided with clinical dexterity include:

- How has practice changed since I first qualified as a midwife?
- Can I practise this skill in other ways?
- How has my previous experience influenced how I approach this procedure today?
- How can I be sure I am carrying this out correctly?
- Are there opportunities for practising this skill elsewhere?
- Who can I observe to explore alternative ways of doing this?

Models of care

A midwife works in many settings and in a range of maternity care systems. For example, she may work independently providing holistic client-centred care, or she may work within a large tertiary centre providing care for women with specific health needs. The models of care can be influential in determining the care that a woman may receive, who from, and when. Midwives need to consider the most appropriate ways that care can be delivered so that they can influence future development in the best interests of women and their families.

Questions that need to be addressed to ensure that the impact of the way

that care is provided is acknowledged include:

- How long has care been provided in this way?
- How is the maternity service organized?
- Which professional groups are involved in the provision of this service?
- How is this procedure/care influenced by the model of care provided?
- How does this model of care impact on the carers?
- How does this model of care impact on the woman and her family?
- Is this the best way to provide care from a professional point of view?

Safe environment

The NMC Code states that 'you must have the skills and knowledge for safe and effective practice when working without direct supervision' (NMC 2008:04). The midwife must ensure that the care she gives does not compromise the safety of women and their families. She must therefore create and maintain a safe working environment at all times, wherever she practises.

Questions that need to be addressed to ensure that the woman's care is provided in a safe environment include:

- Can the woman be assured that her confidentiality will be maintained?
- Does the woman understand the implications of giving her consent to this procedure?
- Are there facilities to ensure that her privacy and dignity are maintained?

- Is there somewhere to wash hands?
- Is there an appropriate place to dispose of waste?
- Is the equipment appropriately maintained and free from contamination?
- Is the space adequate to allow ease of movement around the woman without invading her personal space?
- What are the risks involved in this procedure/care and how have they been addressed?
- Are there any risks to the person undertaking this procedure/care?
- Is this environment safe for others who might come into the room?

Promotes health

Providing care for women and their families presents a unique opportunity to influence the health and wellbeing of the public. Midwives must capitalize on their contacts with women to help them achieve a healthy pregnancy and birth and promote lifestyle choices that will benefit women, babies and families in the future.

Questions that need to be addressed to ensure that the woman's care promotes health include:

- Is this procedure/care going to help her or harm her or her baby in any way?

- What are the opportunities to use this procedure to educate her/her family on healthy behaviours?
- What resources can women and families access to help them make healthy lifestyle choices?
- Has enough time been allocated to this aspect of care to make the most of the opportunities to promote healthy living?
- Who else should I involve to ensure that the woman and her family get the best possible advice in this situation?

The book begins with a chapter focusing on the models of antenatal care. The models of care available and accessed by women can have a significant influence on her experience of pregnancy. The following chapters then use the jigsaw model to explore scenarios from practice. Thus the reader is provided with a structure with which to reflect on her care and that of the multi-professional team in which she works. Each chapter includes a range of activities designed to enable the midwife to contextualize the information within her own practice, applying her continually developing knowledge to her own circumstances. The chapters are written so that they can be accessed without having read the previous ones, although we hope you will find the whole book relevant and thought provoking. Enjoy!

References

Department of Health: *Changing childbirth: Report of the Expert Maternity Group Pt. II; Report of the Expert Maternity Group Pt.1*, London, 1993, Department of Health.

Department of Health: *National Service Framework for children, young people and maternity services. Standard 11. Maternity Services*, London, 2004, Department of Health.

Department of Health: *Maternity matters: choice, access and continuity of care in a safe service*, London, 2007, Department of Health.

National Institute for Health and Clinical Excellence (NICE): *Antenatal care: routine care for the healthy pregnant woman. Clinical guideline 62*, London, 2008, National Collaborating Centre for Women's and Children's Health.

Nursing and Midwifery Council (NMC): *Midwives rules and standards*, London, 2004, NMC.

Nursing and Midwifery Council (NMC): *The code. Standards of conduct, performance and ethics for nurses and midwives*, London, 2008, NMC.

Nursing and Midwifery Council (NMC): *Standards for pre-registration midwifery education*, London, 2009, NMC.

Wickham S: Feminism and ways of knowing. In Stewart M, editor: *Pregnancy, birth and maternity care: feminist perspectives*, Oxford, 2004, Books for Midwives, pp 157–168.

Chapter 2

Models of antenatal care: the options available

Trigger scenario

Joanna is 28 years old and lives with her partner Louis in a second floor flat in the outskirts of London. She works full-time and enjoys reading and cooking in her spare time. Joanna is in good health and was surprised when her normally regular menstrual cycle was interrupted. A pregnancy test bought from the local supermarket confirmed that she was pregnant and she thought long and hard about finding the right way to break the news to Louis. He was shocked, but delighted and this unplanned but very much wanted pregnancy began its nine-month course.

Models of antenatal care

Although it is possible to describe various models of antenatal care, in reality each individual system of healthcare provision will inevitably be a variation on a theme. Within each locality there may be a range of options available to a woman and these may also vary depending on where she lives or on the level of perceived risk her pregnancy presents. Hence the following descriptions provide a broad outline of the main models of care in the United Kingdom rather than an exhaustive list of every permutation available.

Schedules of antenatal care

To appreciate the range of antenatal care provision today it is useful to see it in the context of how care has been organized over the years.

The pattern of antenatal care in the United Kingdom was originally laid down in a Report from the Ministry of Health in 1929. It stated that women should be seen every fortnight from 28 weeks of pregnancy and then weekly from 36 weeks until the baby was born. It is a pattern still familiar to many currently practising midwives. However, this regimented pattern of care was challenged by Hall et al (1980) who concluded that the detection of asymptotic problems during routine antenatal care was low and that the number of visits for low-risk women could be considerably reduced. Sikorski et al (1996) conducted a randomized controlled trial comparing traditional care (13 visits) with 'new style' care (seven visits). The results demonstrated that in reality there was less difference between the mean number of visits that women actually received than anticipated (10.8 visits compared with 8.6 in the study group). They evaluated both clinical outcomes and client satisfaction. No statistical significance was found between clinical outcomes but women were more dissatisfied if they had fewer visits as they valued regular contact with professionals. Midwives also have some reservations about reduced schedules of care, in particular regarding the detection of raised blood pressure and in relation to developing a relationship with the woman (Sanders et al 1999). In a Swedish study (Hildingsson et al 2002) women preferred more antenatal visits if it was their first pregnancy or if they had a previous negative reproductive experience. Older women and those with more than two children preferred fewer visits. The World Health Organization (WHO) has taken a proactive stance regarding the scheduling of antenatal care. In a multi-centre trial involving 24 678 women, a model comprising a screening checklist and a basic package of four antenatal visits was implemented and evaluated (Villar et al 2001). The content of each visit was also specified and outcomes revealed minimal differences between the study and control groups for maternal, fetal and neonatal outcomes (Villar & Bergsjo 2002). The conclusions of this trial are supported by a systematic review of antenatal care for low-risk pregnancies (Villar et al 2008) which again highlighted that maternal satisfaction is often diminished when contact with health professionals is reduced.

Schedules of antenatal care vary between individual Trusts, consultants, midwives and women. Although a general ideal pattern may be part of written guidance for practice, it is appropriate that care reflects the individual needs of women. Since 2003, national guidance has recommended seven antenatal appointments for multiparous women and 10 for primiparous women (NICE 2003; NICE 2008).

Activity

Visit the following website: http://www. who.int/making_pregnancy_safer/ publications/Standards1.6N.pdf

Find Box 1 (p. 3) and consider 'The essential elements of care in pregnancy'. Are they relevant to antenatal care in the UK?

How would they help you provide woman-centred care?

Women will have their own expectations in relation to what antenatal care can do for them. For example, Hildingsson et al (2002) in their study involving 3061 women, reported that women had high expectations of antenatal care in relation to preventing fetal morbidity. Women need to receive realistic information about the care they receive and what the limits of reproductive technologies are.

The following list provides an overview of what antenatal care aims to achieve:

- Diagnose pregnancy and assess the associated risk through evaluation of the woman's previous and current obstetric, medical and social history
- Facilitate the development of a relationship with the woman and her carer that enables effective communication
- Provide evidence-based information about choices for care in a way that is meaningful to the woman and her partner
- Confirm and monitor maternal and fetal wellbeing throughout pregnancy, referring to appropriate specialist help if not within normal limits
- Prepare the woman and her birthing partner for labour and parenthood
- Provide an accessible source of support to pregnant women.

A number of objectives are required in order to meet each of these aims. Many will be generic but some will be specific to the individual needs of each family unit. The content and delivery of antenatal care will be discussed in subsequent chapters in this book.

Activity

Find your copy of the *Midwives rules and standards* (NMC 2004). Find the list of the 'activities of a midwife' (Extract from the EU Second Midwifery Directive 80/155/EEC, Article 4). Read them and identify which apply to your role within antenatal care.

Who provides antenatal care?

In a national survey (Redshaw et al 2007), 49% of women were cared for exclusively by midwives in the antenatal period. Doctors at the hospital were involved in the care of 39% of women, 13% had shared care from a general practitioner (GP) and midwife and 1% of respondents were cared for exclusively by their GP.

Although midwives are able to provide total care to childbearing women, their sphere of practice is normality and they are bound by the *Midwives rules and standards* (NMC 2004) to refer women to an appropriate health professional if her condition deviates from normal (Rule 6). Women will continue to require midwifery care in such circumstances and it is the cooperation and respect between professionals that will enhance the woman's experience of her care.

Midwives

Midwives are the experts in the provision of antenatal care for low-risk women:

The midwife is a person who…works in partnership with women to give the necessary support, care and advice during pregnancy…this care includes preventative measures…the detection of complications in mother and child, the accessing of medical care or other appropriate assistance and the carrying out of emergency measures. The midwife has an important task in health counselling and education…this work should involve antenatal education and preparation for parenthood…

International Confederation of Midwives
(ICM 2005)

This care is often delivered in partnership with either a GP or an obstetrician. The maxim of the government policy document *Maternity matters* (Department of Health 2007a) is that 'all women need a midwife and some need doctors too' (p. 15). However, the role of the midwife as the lead professional for women with uncomplicated pregnancies has been recognized (Department of Health 1993, Department of Health 2007a), if not universally adopted. There is also a move to ensure that all women have access to a midwife as the first point of contact when she confirms her pregnancy (Department of Health 2004, Department of Health 2006, Department of Health 2007a, Department of Health 2007b). Community midwives generally provide the majority of antenatal care to women with uncomplicated pregnancies. This care usually takes place in community health centres or GPs' surgeries and increasingly in children's centres. Within most maternity systems there are midwives who work mostly either in the hospital or community setting, although

some work across both primary and secondary care. Some midwives work independently from the National Health Service (NHS) and are employed by women for a fee, usually fixed. Women who are able to access the services of an independent midwife can then expect continuity of care from a known carer.

Hospital midwives provide care for women attending antenatal clinics for specialist tests and investigations or for monitoring of high-risk pregnancies. Clinics, where consultants from a range of specialisms attend, provide care for pregnant women who also have underlying medical problems. Some hospitals have antenatal day care units where women can attend for assessment and care, without having to stay in hospital. Inevitably a minority of women will need to stay in hospital at some point during their pregnancy and midwives work with obstetricians to plan care that meets their unique needs.

General practitioners

Most women go to their GP when they suspect they are pregnant. Redshaw et al (2007) reported that 83% of respondents presented at their GP when first pregnant and 13% to a midwife. The GP then usually refers the woman to a hospital consultant or the community midwife attached to the practice. However, the continued input of GPs into antenatal care is variable. Research undertaken by Battersby & Thomson (1997) found that no clear parameters emerged when GPs were asked to describe their role in antenatal care. Some maintain or develop a strong interest in obstetrics and continue to see women, perhaps alternating with the midwife, throughout the woman's pregnancy. GPs are uniquely placed to offer care for women and their families over a number of years rather than just a few months (Sikorski et al 1995). However, different priorities, perspectives and geographical locations can contribute to fragmented or duplicated services (Marsh & Renfrew 1999; Renfrew et al 2008).

Consultant obstetricians

Although many women are booked under a particular consultant for their obstetric care, it is unlikely that they will receive much direct care from them, unless they have a high-risk pregnancy. Consultant obstetricians usually have a team of doctors working with them at varying levels of obstetric training, who assist with the management of such women's care. Some consultants also work in private practice.

Specialists

As technology advances, more women are becoming pregnant who would previously have remained childless. Conditions such as cystic fibrosis, diabetes and cardiac anomalies now complicate pregnancies that hitherto would not have been conceived. The care of such women needs to be closely coordinated and monitored and will require a plan of action that involves senior professionals including, for example, paediatricians, anaesthetists

and intensive therapy staff. Care is provided in joint clinics where specialists and obstetricians can work together to provide coordinated woman-centred care.

Social services

Some women will benefit from the additional services provided by social workers, particularly those women whose social circumstances are complicated by poverty, abuse and disadvantage. Such vulnerable women may include: teenage parents, homeless women, victims of domestic violence and substance misuse. It is particularly important that their care is carefully coordinated and that they have a named midwife who has an in-depth insight into their unique history and personal challenges.

Health visitors

The role of the health visitor traditionally focuses on care of families with children under 5 years of age. Although not directly responsible for antenatal care, health visitors often introduce themselves to pregnant women in the antenatal period and may already be involved in monitoring the health and wellbeing of the unborn baby's siblings. In some areas, health visitors also take on a specialist role, for example, supporting teenage parents, and they often contribute to preparation for parenthood classes.

Support workers

Midwives cannot delegate their role to anyone other than a registered medical practitioner (NMC 2004).

However, there are aspects of the midwife's job that can be supported by appropriately trained healthcare support workers, ranging from clerical and housekeeping duties to direct client contact in the promotion of public health (Sandall et al 2007). Maternity support workers, working within clearly defined protocols, are likely to make an increasing contribution to the delivery of maternity services in the future (Department of Health 2007a).

Activity

Next time you care for a woman in late pregnancy, consult her notes and identify how many professionals she has seen during her pregnancy.

What would you think is the minimum number of staff a woman would need to see during the antenatal period?

Models of care

It has been seen that there are a range of healthcare professionals who contribute to the provision of maternity services. Combined with a variety of models of care, the organisation of maternity care is unique to each locality. The last decade has seen a plethora of different schemes designed to meet the recommendations of the document *Changing childbirth* (Department of Health 1993) including more continuity of carer, more community based services and better use of midwives skills. These schemes have often been implemented and evaluated alongside the old or 'traditional' system.

With the availability of so many models of care, it is important that all new services are carefully evaluated to monitor not only the impact on women but also on those providing the service (Campbell & Garcia 1997).

Shared care

A traditional model of antenatal care is when care is shared between the hospital obstetrician and the GP and midwife in primary care. Women may attend the hospital early in pregnancy for their ultrasound scans and then have the majority of their care in the community until the pregnancy is either approaching or post-term, when their pregnancy is reviewed by a hospital doctor. In the traditional model, community midwives work almost exclusively in the primary care setting providing antenatal and postnatal care, with a rota for 24 hour on-call support for home births.

Midwife-led care

In this model of care, midwives are the lead professionals for women who are deemed 'low-risk'. Women who are cared for within this scheme need never see a medical practitioner unless their progress deviates from normal. Criteria for being and remaining low-risk are employed to ensure that there are clear pathways of referral should a woman need to have additional specialist maternity care. Care is usually based entirely in the community, although there are some midwife-led units attached to larger obstetric maternity units, that provide antenatal and postnatal care as well as intrapartum care.

Integrated care

Some obstetric units employ midwives to work in both hospital and community settings within the same working week. This integrated model requires the midwife to be up-to-date with the full repertoire of midwifery skills, as she may be supporting a woman undergoing induction of labour for pre-eclampsia one day and the next be helping another woman express breastmilk at home. Midwives have always been required to be able to practise the whole range of their remit, especially in an emergency. For example, a woman attending antenatal clinic in the community may unexpectedly go into premature labour and the attending community midwife will need to provide competent care and support. This way of working ensures that the maternity unit has a flexible workforce able to meet the unpredictable workload demands of the service. This is particularly important in small units where there may not be a large workforce to rely on if there is a sudden influx of demand or a shortfall of staff. It can be very rewarding for midwives to work in this way but it can also be exhausting to work a mixture of different day and night duties in the same week.

Team midwifery

There are many different ways in which maternity services are organized and deliver a team midwifery approach to care (Wraight et al 1993). The main focus of team midwifery when first introduced was to provide continuity of care from a known carer, hence teams of midwives were created to cover antenatal, intrapartum and postnatal care for a caseload of women. Such teams usually comprise a defined group of midwives who either work from a Primary Care Trust (PCT) in the community, in private practice or from an NHS Hospital Trust. One of the first examples of team midwifery was the 'Know your midwife' scheme which operated in Tooting between 1983 and 1985. Low-risk women were randomized to receive most of their care from one of a team of four midwives, or conventional hospital care (Flint & Poulengeris 1987). The scheme was associated with increased satisfaction with antenatal care and feeling more prepared for parenthood. However, some teams are merely organisational groupings rather than ways of providing continuity for women, and should not be confused with the former. A group of midwives may link with a particular consultant or a geographical location.

Activity

Joanna's last menstrual period (LMP) was 15/8/08. Work out her expected date of delivery (EDD). Find out what models of antenatal care are available in your locality.

Joanna is now 6 weeks pregnant. List five symptoms that she may be experiencing.

Revise how pregnancy is diagnosed.

Check that you know what term is used to describe Joanna's developing baby.

Sure Start

This is the government's programme to integrate health, education and childcare support for families with children under 5 years of age. It is the government's aim to provide this service from children's centres in every community by 2010 (Department of Health 2007c). The aim is that this centre will be a one-stop shop for families to access a range of services and professionals under one roof. Midwives are already integrating into the Sure Start teams and providing antenatal and postnatal support to local women.

Group practice

An example of this innovative model of care is the Albany Midwifery Practice (Reid 2002). It is an independently run, self-managed group of seven midwives and a practice manager contracted into the NHS (hence women do not have to pay for the service). Continuity of carer is offered by two known midwives, throughout the childbirth continuum, although the midwives do not work in fixed pairs. A significant difference between the team and group practice model is that midwives in the latter are only on call for women in their own caseload.

Caseload midwifery

Partnership caseload practice schemes such as the Birth Under Midwifery Practice Scheme (BUMPS) described and evaluated by Benjamin et al (2001) consists of three pairs of midwives. They provide total care to a caseload

of women, attached to a GP practice, with each midwife supporting in labour approximately 40 women per year. Antenatally, women were cared for by the same two midwives throughout their pregnancy. Compared with the traditional model of care, women cared for under BUMPS had more home births, fewer epidurals, more normal births and less induction of labour. They were more likely to go to hospital early and be cared for by a midwife they knew. One-to-one midwifery practice (McCourt & Page 1996) is also a scheme of care whereby each woman (irrespective of risk status) gets to know one midwife, who plans and provides the majority of her care, supported by a second midwife.

Independent midwifery practice

Midwives may practise in a range of settings (ICM 2005) having completed a programme of preparation and gained the requisite qualifications. Some midwives choose to work independently from the NHS and offer a flexible, personalized service to women in their own homes. Sometimes independent midwives work with another midwife for mutual support and on-call cover. Women can contract for all or part of their care depending on their requirements. Independent midwifery in the UK is facing serious threat as the government moves forward with plans to make professional indemnity insurance (PII) a pre-requisite of professional registration. Independent midwives have previously got round their inability to hold insurance by informing women when they contract to care for them, that they do not have PII and what the implication of this might mean. However, the government strategy may make it illegal to practise midwifery without PII.

All midwives, wherever they practise in the UK, must adhere to *Midwives rules and standards* (NMC 2004) and *The Code* (NMC 2008). They must notify their intention to practise to a Supervisor of Midwives in the Local Supervising Authority (LSA) in the area in which they intend to work.

Consultant care

Some women with high-risk pregnancies will need to have their antenatal progress closely supervised by a consultant obstetrician and other senior colleagues. This care will take place at the hospital where there are facilities available for detailed monitoring. However, the woman should still be given the opportunity to develop a relationship with her community midwife who will also support her in the postnatal period.

Activity

Consider each model of care.
What are the implications, the advantages and disadvantages of each model for:

- Women
- Midwives
- Other health professionals
- The Primary Care Trust (PCT) or the Hospital Trust.

Reflection on trigger scenario

Joanna is pregnant for the first time and appears to be in good health. She therefore should be able to choose to have care that meets her needs. It is important that women are given appropriate information when they consider which type of care they want to access. For example, midwives are the experts in normal pregnancy and birth and therefore if a woman does not have any known risk factors, she should be able to access midwife-led care.

Questions that arise from the scenario include:

- How can Joanna find information about who to go to now she knows she is pregnant?
- What information do shop-bought pregnancy tests include about accessing maternity services?
- What provision is there where you work for midwife-led care?
- Can low-risk women go through their entire pregnancy and birth without seeing a medical practitioner?

Conclusion

Joanna has faced the hurdle of telling her partner that they are going to have a baby. She is probably unaware of the many systems and professionals that exist to support her throughout pregnancy. Midwives work in a range of settings with professionals whose roles and skills are complementary. Effective team working and mutual respect will enhance the woman's experience of her care.

Resources

Berg M: Model for high risk antenatal care: a midwifery model of care for childbearing women at high risk: genuine caring in caring for the genuine, *Journal of Perinatal Education* 14(1):9–21, 2005.

Caseload midwifery. Association of Radical Midwives: http://www.midwifery.org.uk/case%20loading.htm.

Home birth reference site: http://www.homebirth.org.uk/.

National Institute for Health and Clinical Excellence: *Antenatal care: routine care for the healthy pregnant woman: Clinical guideline 62*. Online. Available http://www.nice.org.uk/nicemedia/pdf/CG062NICEguideline.pdf, London, 2008, NICE.

One mother one midwife: http://www.onemotheronemidwife.org.uk/evidence.htm.

Sure start: http://www.surestart.gov.uk/.

World Health Organization: Standards for maternal and neonatal care, 2006. Online. Available http://www.who.int/making_pregnancy_safer/publications/standards/en/index.html March 25, 2008.

References

Battersby S, Thomson AM: Community midwives' and general practitioners' perspectives of antenatal care in the community, *Midwifery* 13:92–99, 1997.

Benjamin Y, Walsh D, Taub N: A comparison of partnership caseload midwifery care with conventional team midwifery care: labour and birth outcomes, *Midwifery* 17(3):234–240, 2001.

Campbell R, Garcia J, editors: *The organisation of maternity care: a guide to evaluation*, Hale, 1997, Hochland & Hochland.

Department of Health: *Changing childbirth. Part 1: Report of the Expert Maternity Group*, London, 1993, HMSO.

Department of Health: *National Service Framework for children, young people and maternity services. Standard 11. Maternity Services*, London, 2004, Department of Health.

Department of Health: *Our health, our care, our say*, London, 2006, Department of Health.

Department of Health: *Maternity matters: choice, access and continuity of care in a safe service*, London, 2007a, Department of Health.

Department of Health: (Shribman S) *Making it better: for mother and baby. Clinical case for change*, London, 2007b, Department of Health.

Department of Health: *Delivering health services through Sure Start children's centres*, London, 2007c, Department of Health.

Flint C, Poulengeris P: *The know your midwife report*, London, 1987, South West Thames Regional Health Authority and the Wellington Foundation.

Hall MH, Chng PK, Macgillivray I: Is routine antenatal care worthwhile? *Lancet* 12(7):78–80, 1980.

Hildingsson I, Waldenstrom U, Radestad I: Women's expectations on antenatal care as assessed in early pregnancy: number of visits, continuity of caregiver and general content, *Acta Obstetrica et Gynecologica Scandinavica* 81:118–125, 2002.

International Confederation of Midwives (ICM): *Definition of the midwife*, Brisbane, 2005, ICM. Online. Available http://www.internationalmidwives.org/Portals/5/Documentation/ICM%20Definition%20of%20the%20Midwife%202005.pdf.

Marsh G, Renfrew M: *Community-based maternity care*, Oxford, 1999, Oxford University Press.

McCourt C, Page L, editors: *Report on the evaluation of one to one midwifery practice*, London, 1996, The Hammersmith Hospitals NHS Trust & Thames Valley University.

Ministry of Health: *Maternal mortality in childbirth. Ante-natal clinics: their conduct and scope*, London, 1929, HMSO.

National Institute for Health and Clinical Excellence (NICE): *Antenatal care: routine care for the healthy pregnant woman. Clinical guideline 62*, London, 2003, National Collaborating Centre for Women's and Children's Health.

National Institute for Health and Clinical Excellence (NICE): *Antenatal care: routine care for the healthy pregnant woman. Clinical guideline 62*, London, 2008, National Collaborating Centre for Women's and Children's Health.

Nursing and Midwifery Council (NMC): *Midwives rules and standards*, London, 2004, NMC.

Nursing and Midwifery Council (NMC): *The code. Standards of conduct, performance and ethics for nurse and midwives*, London, 2008, NMC.

Redshaw M, Rowe R, Hockley C, et al: *Recorded delivery: a national survey of women's experience of maternity care*, Oxford, 2007, National Perinatal Epidemiology Unit.

Reid B: The Albany Midwifery Practice, *MIDIRS Midwifery Digest* 14(1): 118–121, 2002.

Renfrew M, Gerrard J, Baston H: Community based maternity care in 2008, *British Journal of General Practice* 58(548):149–150, 2008.

Sandall J, Manthorpe J, Mansfield A, et al: *Support workers in maternity services: a national scoping study of NHS Trusts providing maternity care in England 2006*, London, 2007, King's College.

Sanders J, Somerset M, Jewell D, et al: To see or not to see? Midwives' perceptions of reduced antenatal attendances for low-risk women, *Midwifery* 15(4):257–263, 1999.

Sikorski J, Clement S, Wilson J, et al: A survey of health professionals' views on possible changes in the provision and organisation of antenatal care, *Midwifery* 11:61–68, 1995.

Sikorski J, Wilson J, Clement S, Das S, et al: A randomised controlled trial comparing two schedules of antenatal visits: the antenatal care project, *British Medical Journal* 312(7030):546–553, 1996.

Villar J, Ba'aqeel H, Piaggio G, et al for the WHO Antenatal Care Trial Research Group: WHO antenatal care randomised trial for the evaluation of a new model of routine antenatal care, *The Lancet* 357:1551–1564, 2001.

Villar J, Bergsjo P for the WHO Antenatal Care Trial Research Group: *WHO antenatal care randomised control trial: Manual for the implementation of the new model*, Geneva, 2002, World Health Organization.

Villar J, Carroli G, Khan-Neelofur D, et al: Patterns of routine antenatal care for low-risk pregnancy, *Cochrane Database of Systematic Reviews*, 4(CD000934).

Wraight A, Ball J, Seccombe I, Stock J, et al: *Mapping team midwifery. IMS Report Series 242*, Brighton, 1993, Institute of Manpower Studies.

Chapter 3

The booking history

Trigger scenario

*Joanna is in the first trimester of her
first pregnancy. She has seen her general
practitioner (GP) who gave her some
general advice about what she should
and should not be eating. Aware of her
previous medical history, the GP told
Joanna to go to the reception desk and to
make an appointment for the community
midwife to visit her at home to undertake
the 'booking'. A week later she received a
package of information and a letter from
the midwife confirming the appointment
time and asking Joanna to produce an
early morning specimen of urine (EMSU)
on the day of the visit.*

Introduction

The initial purpose of this important
first appointment with the midwife is
to initiate antenatal care. However, it
should be noted that when the woman
confirms her pregnancy, it is also an
opportunity to provide her with valuable
information, particularly about: folic acid
supplementation, antenatal screening,
nutrition and food hygiene and lifestyle
advice (NICE 2008). If women access
midwifery services directly, rather than
going through a GP, this will enable
them to take earlier advantage of this
opportunity (Department of Health
2007).The information and advice can be
reinforced at the subsequent booking visit.

Depending on the locality and model
of antenatal care practised (see Ch. 2)
the booking history may be conducted
by the community midwife either in
the woman's home or at the local clinic,
or by a midwife at the hospital. It is
usually conducted between 8–12 weeks
of pregnancy, although there is some
evidence that women feel the need for
antenatal care before this time (Sanders
2000). NICE (2008) recommends that
booking is undertaken by 10 weeks of
pregnancy.

The booking visit is probably the
most significant in the pregnancy, and

is an opportunity for the woman and the midwife to get to know each other, as well as meeting the following broad aims to:

- Initiate the development of a trusting relationship between the woman and the midwife
- Present and discuss the options regarding the place of birth
- Present and discuss the options for antenatal screening
- Identify potential risk factors that may complicate the pregnancy through completion of the maternity record
- Identify and agree on an appropriate schedule of antenatal care
- Undertake baseline observations
- Offer lifestyle advice.

We shall explore each in turn.

Developing relationships

Fundamental to all aspects of midwifery care is the need for the midwife to communicate effectively with the woman. There are aspects of the booking that the midwife can influence in order to help make the experience a positive one.

Place of booking

The place where the woman will be most comfortable and able to talk openly about how she feels is probably her own home. There are several advantages to conducting the booking history at the woman's home address.

The balance of power between woman and health professional is more even. The woman is in her own familiar environment, on her own territory, the midwife is a guest. Clinics and hospitals can be daunting places for women to attend. They may be associated with difficult memories, clinical smells and there are often unfamiliar protocols to follow. Of course, many measures have been taken to make such environments more friendly and relaxed, but the privacy and familiarity associated with one's own home cannot be replicated.

It may take longer to book a woman in her own home, as such an event often involves an element of tea-drinking and social chit-chat about the dog/other children/the new kitchen. Time spent by the community midwife during the booking visit getting to know the woman, not just as an individual but as a member of a family and a community, is an investment for future care. Development of trust and mutual respect at the beginning of pregnancy will enable the woman to ask questions and seek advice throughout the childbirth continuum. Worries can be discussed before they become problems. Booking a woman at home enables the midwife to gain a deeper understanding of the woman's social circumstances, who she lives with and how supported she will be by them.

Although undertaking a booking history in the woman's home is perhaps an ideal situation, women should feel they have the choice. Some women wish to keep their pregnancy secret, for whatever reason, and would not welcome the familiar car of the midwife drawing up outside their house.

Information

The woman should be aware of what the meeting is about and what is expected of her, preferably before the meeting takes place. For example, the midwife will be asking her questions about her past medical history asking her if there have been any babies on either side of the family with congenital health problems.

If the woman is expecting to be able to provide such information she can ask her partner if he is aware of any children on his side of the family who have a condition that might be passed on to their baby. She can ask her mother about her own health as a child and if her mother experienced any complications during her pregnancies. The community midwife may have composed a simple, friendly letter of introduction that outlines the content of the booking visit, giving her contact details if the woman needs to clarify anything or make alternative arrangements.

Communication

Midwives care for women from a range of cultural backgrounds and it is vital that they understand each other. Whilst occasionally relatives undertake the role of interpreter until an appropriate link worker can be located, there is no excuse when a pre-planned meeting such as a booking interview is conducted without a skilled interpreter. In a review of the literature in relation to communication and cultural diversity (Robinson 2002) it is apparent that trained interpreters enhance communication.

We tend to get on best with people who show an interest in what we are saying and who appear to be concerned about our welfare. The midwife can demonstrate that she is there to listen to the woman by sitting down with her. If she is standing up this may convey to the woman that she is on the move and has not got time to talk. If the midwife is doing other things at the same time and not looking at the woman, this may suggest to the woman that she is not listening. While it is important that midwives document significant issues, the midwife should put down her pen when the woman is speaking. The midwife can create an opportunity to pick up her pen again, perhaps by reflecting back what the woman has said ('so let me see if I have got this right…') before she writes it down. The woman then knows that the midwife a) had been listening and b) correctly interpreted what was said.

Clinical results should be recorded contemporaneously but the midwife can continue to nod and smile in affirmation that she is still listening or simply say, 'just let me write this down before I forget', to avoid appearing rude. Pressure of work can make it easy to revert to a list of closed questions, as observed in Methven's revealing study (1989). McCourt (2006) describes three styles of communication by midwives during the booking history: professional, providing expertise and guidance; disciplinary, providing expertise and surveillance and partnership which is much more participative and collaborative, following a conversational style rather than a ceremonial order.

Eye contact is an important aspect of showing attention to another. Less gaze is associated with inattention on the part of the listener (Rungapadiachy 1999).

The physical environment is also important. Whilst in a woman's home the midwife cannot start rearranging the furniture but she can make best use of the layout by endeavouring to ensure that there are no physical barriers between them and that they can face each other at the same level.

Discuss place of birth

Women need to be aware of the options available about place of birth before they can make a decision about what might be best for them. Place of birth is a complicated issue and many factors need to be considered before a fully informed decision can be made. The booking visit is an ideal opportunity to raise the issue, to let the woman know that she has a choice, but not necessarily the right time to seek a definitive decision. In some services, for example the Albany Group Practice (Reid 2002) women are not asked to make a decision until they go into labour. In 2005–6 only 2.6% of women had a planned home birth (The Information Centre 2007). The government are committed to ensuring that, by the end of 2009, 'all women will have a choice in where and how they have their baby' (Department of Health 2007:09).

Although many midwives freely offer choice regarding place of birth, some do not. This may be due to a range of reasons including lack of confidence due to infrequent demand. Some midwives feel that they are not supported by their colleagues (Baston & Green 2002). A midwife may work in a team where the other midwives would not be able to cover her clinic or visits if she was called to a home birth. Crises of low staffing levels sometimes lead units to temporarily withdraw home birth as an option.

Home birth presents the ideal scenario of one to one care in labour for low-risk women. A woman booked for a hospital birth may be cared for by a midwife who is also looking after other women at the same time. However, it would be inappropriate for all women to give birth at home as there are limited options for pharmacological methods of pain relief and many women, especially those experiencing their first labour, wish to have an epidural (Leighton & Halpern 2002). Others have or develop complications either during their pregnancy or birth that preclude home birth as a suitable option as they require the facilities of an obstetric unit and medical or surgical support.

Women need to be aware of the risks and benefits of the options they choose and while we are often quick to raise the risks associated with home birth we are seldom forthright in presenting the risks associated with birth in a hospital environment.

Activity

List the advantages and disadvantages that you perceive might be associated with both hospital and home birth. Think about what obstetric complications might result in a woman being advised to give birth in hospital.

Discuss antenatal screening

The booking interview is often the time when women are given information about the options available to them regarding antenatal screening for fetal abnormality. They may have already heard about some of the tests, through relatives or friends. However, women need to make choices that are right for them as individuals and may require support and guidance about the risks and benefits of the test on offer. The midwife needs to be able to present the facts, without prejudice or personal influence.

The midwife 'should enable the woman to make decisions about her care based on her individual needs,

by discussing matters fully with her' (NMC 2004:17).

The range of tests available varies from locality to locality, and may change as new tests become available. Keeping up-to-date with all the tests on offer presents a challenge to midwives, as they need to know what the test involves, when it is performed, how it is obtained and what the results mean. They also have to be able to translate this into meaningful information for women of all cultures and backgrounds. Keeping abreast of changes in clinical practice is a midwife's professional responsibility (NMC 2008:09).

All women have the right to this information. If a test can only be undertaken through a private company and requires payment, it is not for the midwife to decide if a woman of low socio-economic status should have it or not. Women may face dilemmas about the choices they make, but they cannot address them unless they know that the choices exist. Midwives may have their assumptions challenged with regard to who will benefit from information (Kirkham et al 2002). See Chapter 8 for information about the screening tests available.

Activity

Find out what screening tests are offered for women who book at the Trust where you work. Find out if they are offered to all women or to women in particular categories.

Risk assessment

Taking a booking history is an opportunity to undertake a risk assessment of the pregnancy, as recommended by recent confidential enquiries into maternal death (Lewis 2004; Lewis 2007). In the latest report it was highlighted that there were some cases where midwifery-led care had been provided to women who were known to be high-risk. The use of risk assessment tools varies between maternity services, and their previous value has been questioned, especially for first pregnancies (Enkin et al 2000). It is part of government policy that 'each woman should undergo a standardised risk and needs assessment to help in her decision making process' (Department of Health 2007:14). It is part of the National Institute for Health and Clinical Excellence (NICE 2008) remit to develop an 'antenatal assessment tool' with the proviso that it must be subjected to a multi-centred validation study with the aim of identifying a third of women who are at increased risk of maternal death.

Completion of the maternity record

The national maternity records used for antenatal care encourage the woman to contribute to and be directly involved in her care. There are sections that she can complete herself and identify any questions she might have. As she holds the records throughout the pregnancy she has the opportunity to read them in intimate detail. It is important, therefore, that whenever the midwife makes an entry in the records she explains it to the woman and ensures that she knows not only what it says but also what it means. A systematic review to evaluate the effects of women carrying their own case notes during pregnancy concluded that this system improves women's feeling of control, satisfaction and the availability of antenatal records (Brown & Smith 2004).

Personal information

The national maternity record begins with an important section which the woman can complete herself. It includes details about her full name and title, and what she likes to be called. There are important contact details, essential for the return of lost records, and boxes to record the names of the professionals involved in the woman's maternity care.

It is on this page that the woman also records her occupation and that of the baby's father. This is important information as there may be occupational hazards associated with particular kinds of work that the midwife can give general advice about. Women may need to be encouraged to talk to their employer about reassignment of duties during their pregnancy, depending on the nature of their role. For example, if their job involves heavy lifting or standing for long periods, an alternative office role might be available during the term of the pregnancy.

Previous medical history

This section may also be completed by the woman. It asks the woman to indicate whether she has suffered from any of a list of illnesses. Box 3.1 provides a summary of the potential significance of each condition.

Box 3.1 Health history

- **Anaesthetic problems**
Significance   Previous failed intubation would require the presence of a consultant anaesthetist if caesarean section was needed

- **Asthma or chest problem**
Significance   Needs careful assessment prior to the use of inhalational analgesia or surgery

- **Back problem**
Significance   May need assessment prior to insertion of epidural analgesia

- **Blood transfusion**
Significance   May have developed antibodies in response to previous transfusion

- **Diabetes**
Significance   Will need antenatal care coordinated between medical and obstetric team. Diabetes associated with neonatal morbidity (Seidel et al 1997)

- **Epilepsy**
Significance   Teratogenic risk from anticonvulsant therapy (Crawford 2002). Risk of drowning during seizures (CEMD 2001)

- **Fertility problems**
Significance   May require more frequent attendance at antenatal clinic for reassurance and support

- **Vaginal infections**
Significance   Ascending infection may result in premature labour and/or neonatal morbidity

- **Heart problems**
Significance   May require specialist antenatal and intrapartum care. Increased circulatory volume in pregnancy could compromise cardiopulmonary system

- **High blood pressure**
Significance   More likely to develop pre-eclampsia, therefore needs additional monitoring in pregnancy

- **Kidney or urinary problems**
Significance   Effect of progesterone in pregnancy leads to convolution of ureters, urinary stasis and thus increased potential for urinary tract infection [UTI] (Chamberlain & Morgan 2002). UTI linked with increased risk of premature labour

- **Liver disease or hepatitis**
Significance   Cholestatis may worsen during pregnancy in women with primary biliary cirrhosis

- **Mental health problems**
Significance   History of depression associated with increased risk of postnatal depression. Suicide significant cause of maternal death (CEMD 2001; Lewis 2004)

continued

Box 3.1 Continued

• **Operations**

Significance   For example, cervical surgery may impact on decisions regarding mode of birth; breast surgery may affect ability to breastfeed, etc.

• **Psychological difficulties**

Significance   May impact on ability to cope with the stress of pregnancy or undertake parenting role

• **Thrombosis**

Significance   Needs prophylactic anticoagulation therapy during pregnancy and special monitoring

• **Taken folic acid?**

Significance   0.4 mg folic acid daily pre-conceptually and during pregnancy in the first trimester recommended to reduce the risk of neural tube defects by 75% (MRC Vitamin Study Research Group 1991).

Current medical history

Women may become pregnant with an underlying medical disorder. Often, women confirm their pregnancy with their GP first, hence the woman's medical condition is already known. For example, if the woman has diabetes, the GP would refer the woman directly to a clinic that caters for pregnant women with medical conditions. These clinics have different names, such as 'joint care clinic', where arrangements are made for both the medical team and the obstetric team to see the woman at the same time. Thus care is planned and coordinated to meet the needs of the pregnant woman in the light of her underlying medical condition. Individual maternity services may have alternative systems in place to support the care of local women.

The midwife needs to ascertain the woman's current health status in order to identify any potential problem that might impact on either the woman's or the baby's health. Normal health is a very subjective concept. For example, a woman who usually uses her asthma inhaler four times a day might consider her health to be very good if she has only needed to use it twice a day for the last week. Thus a question such as: 'Are you normally well?' might elicit a positive response. An alternative might be: 'Tell me about your general health – are you currently receiving treatment for anything?' It is important to note any medication currently taken (prescribed, illegal, or over-the-counter) to ensure that nothing is being taken that could potentially harm the developing fetus. It is also important at this point to document any known allergies to drugs or other substances. If the woman is less than 12 weeks' pregnant the midwife should recommend that she takes folic acid, 400 micrograms daily, to reduce the risk of the baby having a neural tube defect.

The National Institute for Health and Clinical Excellence recommends that women aged under 25 years should be informed of the high prevalence of chlamydia in their age group. They should be directed to local screening services (NICE 2008), but chlamydia screening should not form part of routine antenatal care. NICE do not recommend that women are screened routinely for beta-haemolytic Streptococcus. If they are known to have had a previous infection, local policy should be followed.

Activity

Find out about the implications for the unborn baby of being infected with beta-haemolytic Streptococcus.

Identify five drugs that may have a teterogenic effect.

Describe five jobs which might be hazardous during pregnancy and why.

Social history

The woman experiences her pregnancy within a social context. This environment may impact on the health of both the woman and her baby. There are many issues to consider, including social support, financial and housing difficulties. The midwife will need to recognize potential problems and refer the woman to appropriate agencies for specialist help if needed. The following issues are of particular concern:

- *Smoking*: It is widely acknowledged that smoking in pregnancy has significant sequelae for the developing fetus, the mother (Bardy et al 1993) and the child (Haberg et al 2007). Women who smoke expect health professionals to raise the issue, and failure to do so may result in the woman concluding that the professional is unsure of the facts (Haugland et al 1996). There are many schemes and initiatives designed to help pregnant smokers quit the habit, although their effectiveness needs careful evaluation to identify the most appropriate intervention (Hajek et al 2001).

- *Alcohol*: The midwife documents the number of units of alcohol consumed by the woman each week. This provides the opportunity to answer any questions that the issue of alcohol consumption raises and also to provide general guidance. Excessive alcohol consumption can potentially lead to fetal alcohol syndrome, resulting in a range of physical and mental sequalae. The level of safe drinking for pregnant women remains a controversial issue. The Food Standards Agency (2008) recommends abstinence or no more than one or two units, once or twice a week.

- *Domestic violence*: According to a Swedish study (Stenson et al 2001), most women do not object to being asked by their midwife about domestic abuse, including those who have reported exposure to violence.

It is important that the midwife has received education about the issues surrounding domestic violence and that local guidance supports her actions when abuse is disclosed.

Family history

Again, this section in the national maternity records encourages the woman to identify for herself any relevant family history, including diabetes, sickle cell anaemia, thalassaemia, learning disabilities, congenital abnormalities and consanguinity. It is important to identify conditions that may have

relevance to this pregnancy, either in terms of the need for specialist referral or to allay unwarranted fears.

Previous obstetric history

It is important to pay particular attention to a woman's previous experiences. These memories may contribute to how she feels about the forthcoming birth of this baby. It may be an opportunity to clarify misconceptions and address concerns.

For each birth, all the aspects listed in Table 3.1 should be documented.

Taking an accurate previous obstetric history will help highlight factors that

Table 3.1 Previous obstetric history

Type of birth	
Date	
Gestation	
Birth weight	
Place of birth	
Child's name	
Boy/girl	
Age now	

Problems?	No	Yes	Details
During pregnancy			
During the birth			
After the birth			
Baby at birth			
Health now			

might warrant the women being referred for consultant opinion. For example, women who have had a previous low birthweight baby should be closely monitored and offered serial ultrasound scans to identify potential sub-optimum growth in the pregnancy. Being aware of previous events such as emergency caesarean birth, premature labour, antepartum or postpartum haemorrhage, previous small or large baby, pre-eclampsia and gestational diabetes will enable the midwife to plan appropriate and individualized antenatal care.

Box 3.1 outlines the significance of each aspect of the woman's health history in terms of her pregnancy and birth.

Activity

Find out what is meant by parity.
  Write down your description of a woman, in obstetric terms, who was pregnant for the third time, having had one live child and a miscarriage at 10 weeks?

Current obstetric history

It is important to assess how the woman is feeling. So much of the focus so far has been on related issues rather than this pregnancy. The midwife will ask what symptoms of pregnancy the woman has experienced and how she feels generally about being pregnant. She will also establish the first day of the woman's last menstrual period (LMP) and from this work out the woman's expected date of delivery (EDD) (Table 3.2).

Table 3.2 Calculating expected date of delivery

First day of last menstrual period (LMP)	21/8/08
Add one year	21/8/09
Add 7 days	28/8/09
Take away 3 months	28/5/09
EDD=	28/5/09

This calculation is based on a 28-day menstrual cycle. It is important that the midwife establishes what was normal for the woman: how often she bled and for how long. She will ask if the last period was a 'normal' period, as occasionally women experience a small blood loss (nidation) when the fertilized ovum (blastocyst) embeds in the endometrium. As this occurs at approximately the same time as the next period might have been anticipated, it can occasionally be incorrectly perceived as such. If there are uncertainties about the LMP, the EDD may be confirmed by an ultrasound scan (USS), with the woman's consent.

Activity

The first day of Joanna's last menstrual period (LMP) was 21/8/08. Calculate her EDD. Be sure that you can make these calculations using both a calendar and a gestation calculator (wheel). What percentage of babies are born on their EDD?

Table 3.3 BMI classification (WHO 2006)

Underweight	BMI < 18.5
Desirable	BMI 18.5–24.9
Overweight	BMI 25.0–29.9
Obese	BMI > 30
Morbidly obese	BMI > 40

Physical characteristics

Weight is not routinely monitored throughout pregnancy (NICE 2008) by healthcare professionals (although it may be by the pregnant women), but it is important to establish a baseline.

Body mass index (BMI) or the ratio of weight in kilogrammes to height in metres squared, is a useful determinant of obesity (Frolich 2002).

The World Health Organization has recognized five categories of BMI (2006) (see Table 3.3).

Increasing BMI is associated with gestational diabetes, hypertension, thromboembolism and anaesthetic risk, and should be calculated at booking (NICE 2008). The Confidential Enquiries into Maternal Deaths (Lewis 2007) highlighted that over half of the women who died in the triennium 2003–2005 were obese (BMI over 25) and 8% were morbidly obese. The midwife should then follow local guidance regarding referral to a dietician for appropriate assessment and monitoring, once obesity is diagnosed.

Age is also recorded, as extremes of the childbearing continuum are associated with adverse obstetric outcomes. A systematic review of the literature in relation to obstetric outcomes for women aged over 35 years (Palles 2008) concluded that such women had an increased risk of pre-term birth, induction and augmentation of labour, epidural analgesia and operative birth. Women aged over 40 years have an increased risk of pre-eclampsia and more frequent monitoring of blood pressure and urinalysis for proteinurea throughout pregnancy should be considered (NICE 2008).

Clinical observations

The midwife will test the woman's urine for protein and glucose and take her blood pressure, both routine aspects of subsequent antenatal care (NICE 2008). A midstream specimen of urine should also be sent to the laboratory for culture to test for the presence of asymptomatic bacteriuria (NICE 2008) as treatment can prevent pylonephritis, a potentially serious kidney infection. It is also important that an abdominal palpation is undertaken at this time, to pick up advancing or multiple pregnancy, as the uterus is not normally palpable above the symphysis pubis until approximately 12 weeks' gestation.

Blood will also be taken to check Joanna's blood group and rhesus factor, check for anaemia, HIV, syphilis and haemoglobin-opathies (see Ch. 7).

Information giving

It is recommended that women take vitamin D supplement of

10 micrograms of vitamin D each day during pregnancy (NICE 2008). Vitamin D is made by the body through exposure to sunlight and is essential for the development of healthy bones. It has also been reported that vitamin D deficiency increases the risk of pre-eclampsia (Bodnar et al 2007).

NICE guidelines (2008) also recommend that women receive information at booking about how the baby develops during pregnancy, nutrition and diet and exercise, including pelvic floor exercises. They also suggest that women are informed about antenatal classes, maternity benefits, breastfeeding workshops.

Plan appropriate antenatal care

The midwife has collected a wealth of information about the woman's previous and current health status. Local policy will dictate the course of action for women identified as either high- or low-risk, who should be their lead professional and how often they should be seen. National guidance from the National Institute for Health and Clinical Excellence (NICE 2008) recommends 10 appointments for nulliparous women and 7 for parous women. Women will continue to need support from their community midwife, even if they are having specialist consultant care. The plan of action should be discussed and agreed with the woman and then documented in her maternity records.

Reflection on trigger scenario

Look back at the trigger scenario.

Joanna is in the first trimester of her first pregnancy. She has seen her general practitioner who gave her some general advice about what she should and should not be eating. Aware of her previous medical history, the GP told Joanna to go to the reception desk and to make an appointment for the community midwife to visit her at home to undertake the 'booking'. A week later she received a package of information and a letter from the midwife confirming the appointment time and asking Joanna to produce an early morning specimen of urine (EMSU) on the day of the visit.

This scenario presents a traditional model of care whereby the woman goes to her GP to confirm her pregnancy before accessing midwifery care. As the GP has access to her medical notes s/he deems her to be 'low-risk' and therefore refers her to the community midwife for her booking history. Now that you are familiar with the purpose and content of the booking visit, you should have insight into how the scenario reflects current practice. The jigsaw model will now be used to explore the trigger scenario in more depth.

Effective communication

Effective verbal and non-verbal communication is essential in the provision of effective maternity care. Joanna has been to see her GP who also gave her information about healthy eating in pregnancy. Questions that arise from the scenario might include: Did the GP explain the rationale behind the advice s/he gave? Was the information backed up by written information? Was written information supported by a verbal explanation? What methods of communication are there between the receptionist and the midwife and how long does it take for the midwife to become alert to a new pregnancy? What information did Joanna receive through the post? Would it be referred to during the booking interview?

Woman-centred care

Providing personalized care centred around the woman's individual circumstances is central to current maternity policy. Questions that arise from the scenario might include: Did the GP offer Joanna any options for care? Was there time during the consultation with the GP for Joanna to ask specific questions? Were there any specific risk factors associated with Joanna's medical or family history that made her at risk in any way? Was the letter from her midwife personal to Joanna's circumstances or routine? Had Joanna already given an EMSU for laboratory analysis?

Using best evidence

Providing women with information that is based on best evidence enables them to make informed decisions and take an active role in their care.

Questions that arise from the scenario might include: Was the GP aware of the latest national guidance from the National Institute for Health and Clinical Excellence? How is this information disseminated to all health professionals involved in maternity care? Are national guidelines discussed at a local level and previous care pathways amended in their light? What is the evidence about the most appropriate times to give women information? Why is it important to detect asymptomatic bacteriuria?

Professional and legal issues

Midwives must practice within a professional and legal framework to ensure that they protect the women they care for from potential harm and maintain high standards of care. Questions that arise from the scenario might include: Did the GP ask Joanna's consent to refer her to the community midwife? Can the midwife ask the practice nurse to undertake the booking visit? What must the midwife do if she detects an abnormality in Joanna's pregnancy? How is the midwife keeping up-to-date with changes in antenatal care?

Team working

Joanna has already been in contact with four people in relation to her pregnancy: the pharmacist who did her pregnancy test, the GP receptionist who made her GP appointment and who referred her to the midwife, the GP and the midwife by letter. Questions that arise from the scenario might include: How can team working in primary care be enhanced? What might the consequences be for Joanna if the midwife did not receive her referral? What might the consequences be for the midwife? Has the GP provided relevant information to the midwife about Joanna's past and current health status? What mechanisms are there for the community midwife to continue to keep the GP informed of her progress?

Clinical dexterity

Part of the booking visit includes abdominal palpation, blood pressure measurement, urinalysis and venepuncture. All of these clinical observations and procedures require clinical dexterity, confidence and competence. Questions that arise from the scenario might include: How did the midwife learn how to take blood and how was this assessed? Where does the midwife undertake an abdominal palpation in a woman's home? What equipment does the midwife use to take a woman's blood pressure in the home? How does this differ from the equipment the GP might use? What would the midwife do if she could not get a blood sample from Joanna after two attempts?

Models of care

There are many models of care ranging from midwife-led to consultant-led antenatal care. The midwife is responsible for informing woman of her options and enabling her to make the most appropriate choice for her individual circumstances. It is not stated in the scenario how this was discussed

with Joanna. Questions that arise from the scenario might include: What is the full range of options for antenatal care in your locality? What factors influence the model of care chosen? How might the model of care chosen influence the outcome of pregnancy?

Safe environment

It is essential that the midwife takes appropriate precautionary measures when providing clinical care to women. These include ensuring that the environment does not pose a risk to either the woman or herself and following clinical procedures with care. Questions that arise from the scenario might include: Did the midwife wear gloves to take blood from Joanna? How did the midwife dispose of the urine dipstick? When did the midwife wash her hands? How did the midwife dispose of the needle used for venepuncture? How did the midwife check Joanna's personal details for labelling the specimens?

Promotes health

When the woman contacts the GP or midwife at the beginning of pregnancy, it provides her carers with an ideal opportunity to give her information to enable her to make informed healthcare choices. Joanna had already had input from the GP about healthy eating and then information from the midwife through the post, prior to the booking visit. Questions that arise from the scenario might include: What information should the woman receive before her booking history is taken? What advice can the midwife give at booking that will promote Joanna's health during the pregnancy and throughout motherhood? What facilities are there where you work to support a pregnant woman who wishes to stop smoking?

Further scenarios

The following scenarios enable you to consider how specific situations influence the care the midwife provides. Use the jigsaw model to explore the issues raised in each scenario.

Scenario 1

Mary is a 43-year-old mother of two grown-up children who discovers she is pregnant. She is recently divorced and is seeing a man she does not intend staying with. She is unsure about whether to continue with her pregnancy and goes to the GP for advice. He refers her to the community midwife for a home booking visit.

Practice point

Further questions specific to Scenario 1 include:

1. Has the GP asked Mary if she wants to continue with the pregnancy?
2. How would you tactfully approach this issue?
3. Is a home booking appropriate in these circumstances?
4. What systems are in place to offer choice to women regarding where the booking interview takes place?
5. What advice and information might the midwife offer Mary?

6. How do you feel about termination of pregnancy in these circumstances?

Scenario 2

Jessica is 6 weeks pregnant and keen to have a home birth. She makes an appointment directly with the midwife to discuss how to go about this.

Practice point

Further questions specific to Scenario 2 include:

1. What is the optimum time to discuss place of birth?
2. How can the midwife support Jessica in her aspirations?
3. In what circumstances would the midwife recommend that Jessica has a hospital birth?
4. Should parity influence the decision in any way?
5. What advice can the midwife offer Jessica to help her achieve a home birth?

Conclusion

The booking interview presents a unique opportunity for the woman and midwife to form a relationship and develop mutual respect. It may be the first time that the woman has come across a midwife and she may be unclear about her role and what to expect from antenatal care. Ideally she will come away feeling that she has met someone who is competent and caring and with whom she can discuss her hopes and fears.

Resources

Department of Health: http://www.dh.gov.uk/en/index.htm.

Fetal alcohol syndrome aware UK: http://www.fasaware.co.uk/.

Home birth: http://www.homebirth.org.uk/.

National Chlamydia Screening Programme: www.chlamydiascreening.nhs.uk.

NICE Antenatal care guideline 2008-03-28: http://www.rcog.org.uk/resources/public/pdf/Antenatal_care.pdf.

NICE Maternal and Child nutrition guideline: http://www.nice.org.udk/nicemedia/pdf/PH011guidance.pdf.

Smoking in pregnancy: http://smokefree.nhs.uk/questions/smoking-and-pregnancy/.

Sure Start: http://www.surestart.gov.uk/.

References

Bardy AH, Seppala T, Lillsunde P, et al: Objectively measured tobacco exposure during pregnancy: neonatal effects and relation to maternal smoking, *British Journal of Obstetrics and Gynaecology* 100(8):721–726, 1993.

Baston HA, Green JM: Community midwives' role perceptions, *British Journal of Midwifery* 10(1):35–40, 2002.

Bodnar L, Catov J, Simhan H, et al: Maternal vitamin D deficiency increases the risk of pre-eclampsia, *Journal of Endocrinology and Metabolism* 92(9):3517–3522, 2007.

Brown HC, Smith HJ: Giving women their own case notes to carry during pregnancy, *Cochrane Database of Systematic Reviews*, Issue 2, Art. No.: CD002856, 2004.

Chamberlain G, Morgan M: *ABC of antenatal care*, ed 4, London, 2002, BMJ Books.

Confidential Enquiry into Maternal Deaths (CEMD): *Why mothers die 1997–1999. The fifth report of the confidential enquiry into maternal deaths in the United Kingdom*, London, 2001, RCOG.

Crawford P: Epilepsy and pregnancy, *MIDIRS Midwifery Digest* 12(3):327–331, 2002.

Department of Health: *Maternity matters: choice, access and continuity of care in a safe service*, London, 2007, Department of Health.

Enkin M, Keirse MJNC, Neilson J, et al: *A guide to effective care in pregnancy and childbirth*, ed 3, Oxford, 2000, Oxford University Press.

Food Standards Agency: When you are pregnant. Online. Available http://www.eatwell.gov.uk/agesandstages/pregnancy/whenyrpregnant/?lang=en April 27, 2008.

Frolich J: Obesity in pregnancy, *MIDIRS Midwifery Digest* 12(1):39–43, 2002.

Haberg S, Stigum H, Nystad W, et al: Effects of pre- and postnatal exposure to parental smoking on early childhood respiratory health, *American Journal of Epidemiology* 166(6):679–686, 2007.

Hajek P, West R, Lee A, et al: Randomised controlled trial of a midwife-delivered brief: smoking cessation intervention in pregnancy, *Addiction* 96(3):485–494, 2001.

Haugland S, Haug K, Wold B: A pregnant smoker's experience of antenatal care: results from a qualitative study, *Scandinavian Journal of Primary Health Care* 14(4):216–222, 1996.

Kirkham M, Stapleton H, Curtis P, et al: Stereotyping as a professional defence mechanism, *British Journal of Midwifery* 10(9):549–552, 2002.

Leighton BL, Halpern SH: The effects of epidural analgesia on labor, maternal and neonatal outcomes: a systematic review, *American Journal of Obstetrics and Gynaecology* 186(5):S69–S77, 2002.

Lewis G, editor: *Confidential enquiry into maternal and child health. Improving the health of mothers, babies and children. Why mothers die 2000–2002. Midwifery summary and key recommendations,* London, 2004, RCOG.

Lewis G, editor: *Confidential enquiry into maternal and child health (CEMACH). Saving mothers' lives: reviewing maternal deaths to make motherhood safer – 2003–2005. The seventh report on confidential enquiries into maternal deaths in the United Kingdom,* London, 2007, CEMACH.

McCourt C: Supporting choice and control? Communication and interaction between midwives and women at the antenatal booking visit, *Social Science & Medicine* 62:1307–1318, 2006.

Methven E: Recording an obstetric history or relating to pregnant women? A study of the antenatal booking interview. In Robinson S, Thomson AM, editors: *Midwives, research and childbirth,* (vol I), London, 1989, Chapman and Hall.

MRC Vitamin Study Research Group: Prevention of neural tube defects: results of the Medical Research Council vitamin study, *Lancet* 338(8760):131–137, 1991.

National Institute for Health and Clinical Excellence (NICE): *Antenatal care: routine care for the healthy pregnant woman. Clinical guideline 62,* London, 2008, National Collaborating Centre for Women's and Children's Health.

Nursing and Midwifery Council (NMC): *Midwives rules and standards,* London, 2004, NMC.

Nursing and Midwifery Council (NMC): *The code. Standards of conduct, performance and ethics for nurses and midwives,* London, 2008, NMC.

Palles K: Advancing maternal age: a risk indicator or risk factor for primiparous women in childbearing? A systematic review, *MIDIRS Midwifery Digest* 18(1):7–18, 2008.

Reid B: The Albany Midwifery Practice, *MIDIRS Midwifery Digest* 14(1):118–121, 2002.

Robinson M: *Communication and health in a multi-ethnic society*, Bristol, 2002, Policy Press.

Rungapadiachy DM: *Interpersonal communication and psychology for the health care professional: theory and practice*, Oxford, 1999, Butterworth-Heinemann.

Sanders J: Let's start at the very beginning…Women's comments on early pregnancy care, *MIDIRS Midwifery Digest* 10(2):169–173, 2000.

Seidel HM, Rosensein BJ, Pathak A: *Primary care of the newborn*, ed 2, St Louis, 1997, Mosby.

Stenson K, Saarinen H, Heimer G, et al: Women's attitudes to being asked about exposure to violence, *Midwifery* 17(1):2–10, 2001.

The Information Centre: NHS Maternity Statistics, England: 2005–2006, The Information Centre, 2007. Online. Available http://www.ic.nhs.uk/webfiles/publications/maternity0506/NHSMaternityStatsEngland200506_fullpublication%20V3.pdf.

World Health Organization: BMI classification, 2006. Online. Available http://www.who.int/bmi/index.jsp?introPage=intro_3.html. March 26, 2008.

Chapter 4

Health in pregnancy

Trigger scenario

Joanna is now 20 weeks pregnant. She has been well, although rather nauseous at times, but this is now less frequent. She gave up smoking 3 weeks ago and is now beginning to struggle. She even got to the stage where she took one of Louis' cigarettes from the packet and searched through the kitchen drawer to find a lighter that worked. She was interrupted by an interesting text message and then managed to gather her willpower to put the cigarette back in its packet.

Introduction

Pregnancy is not an illness, but a time of changing physiology and great anticipation. This chapter will focus on factors that impact on both the woman's health and that of her developing baby. Issues that relate specifically to emotional wellbeing and mental health will be considered in Chapter 6.

There are many sources of information available for women regarding achieving a healthy pregnancy. They are produced by government agencies, commercial businesses, local trusts, user and support groups and professional bodies. Some women experience very few problems in relation to their health, have a spontaneous labour and give birth to a healthy baby, without making any conscious changes to their usual way of life. However, many women seek and require advice about the physical and emotional changes they experience, and look to the midwife for support and the provision of effective information.

Health in pregnancy

One rationale for achieving a healthy lifestyle during pregnancy is to maximize the likelihood of having a healthy baby and to avoid inadvertently harming the baby by being unaware of potentially hazardous behaviour. Women need information so that they can make decisions about how they can alter or adapt their lifestyle. It is not currently a criminal offence in the United Kingdom for a woman to potentially put her baby at risk, for example, by smoking or drinking alcohol during pregnancy. However, it is part of the midwife's role to advise women during pregnancy and offer health counselling and education (ICM 2005). To fail to inform a woman of known potential risks to her or her baby's health would be to breach the midwife's duty of care. The midwife therefore needs to have a working knowledge of how women can optimize their health, for the benefit of both their own and their baby's wellbeing.

Diet

The issue of what pregnant women eat has generated much discussion over the years. Aspects of debate include the quantity and quality of food, and pregnancy-associated changes to women's dietary intake. It has been reported that maternal nutrition during pregnancy may have a significant impact on future adult health (Barker 1992).

Quantity

Although it is not part of routine antenatal care to weigh women every time they attend clinic (NICE 2008), many women do keep an eye on their own weight gain. There is a wide range of weight gain associated with normal outcome; however, average weight gain for mothers of full-term babies is 11–15 kg (Stables & Rankin 2005). The pregnant woman has additional nutritional requirements, including increased calorific intake (300 kcal daily), increased protein (6 g daily), folate supplementation (400 µg daily) and increased dietary calcium and iron (Coad 2001).

Severe dietary restriction can result in significant reduction in birthweight (Enkin et al 2000). The NICE guidance on improving nutrition for pregnant and breastfeeding mothers (NICE

2008) highlights the prevalence of malnutrition, particularly in low-income households, with one-fifth of adults having small meals or skipping them altogether. Women with low incomes are eligible for Healthy Start vouchers to enable them to buy fruit and vegetables (Department of Health 2004). A systematic review (Kramer 2000) found that dietary supplementation with both calories and protein resulted in both maternal weight gain and increased birthweight with a subsequent decrease in small for gestational age infants and lower perinatal mortality. The same review concluded that restricting the energy or protein intake of obese women may be harmful.

Obesity in pregnancy is associated with increased obstetric risk, including gestational diabetes, hypertension, operative intervention, anaesthetic complications, prolonged labour and shoulder dystocia (Frohlich 2002). There is also evidence that maternal obesity is associated with an increased risk of fetal abnormality (Watkins et al 2003). In the Confidential Enquiry into maternal death 2003–2005 (Lewis 2007) it was reported that over 50% of women who died were overweight, compared with 35% in the previous triennium (Lewis 2004). Although women are often advised not to lose weight in pregnancy (Food Standards Agency 2008a), this may be a time when they are receptive to nutritional advice (Richens 2008). A systematic review of the benefits of a low glycaemic diet in pregnancy to reduce the risks of gestational diabetes mellitus (Tieu et al 2008) concluded that although

the results suggested this to be beneficial, the evidence was not strong enough to be conclusive. Claesson et al (2008) report on a case control intervention study of motivational talks and aquarobic exercise classes for obese women. Although the intervention was not associated with any difference between the groups for obstetric variables, the intervention group had significantly less weight gain during pregnancy than the control group. Women with a BMI over $30 \, kg/m^2$ should be referred for consultant care (Richens 2008) and screened for diabtetes (NICE 2008). Those women with a BMI over $35 \, kg/m^2$ should be considered for aspirin therapy, in the presence of additional risk factors for pre-eclampsia, and for thromboprophylaxis if they have additional risk factors for thromboembolic disease (RCOG 2007).

Quality

Women are faced with an increasing range of foods that they are advised not to eat when pregnant, because of the potential risk to the developing fetus. There are also many supplements available over the counter for women who are pregnant or considering pregnancy.

Soft cheese, unpasteurised dairy products and paté

These foods are associated with the bacteria known as *Listeria monocytogenes*. All fruit and vegetables should be washed before eating as the bacteria is found in soil. The bacteria is killed by heat and women should be advised to ensure that all meats are cooked thoroughly and that takeaway food is eaten piping hot (Food Standards Agency 2008a). The infection may present as flu-like symptoms in the pregnant women and can be transferred to the fetus via the placenta or during the birth. When contracted before birth the baby may develop septicaemia, with an associated mortality rate of 30%, although this is reduced if the infection is confirmed and antibiotic therapy is given. If the baby contracts the infection following the birth the outlook is better (Seidel et al 1997). Offensive liquor and placental cysts may have alerted the midwife to suspect infection, initiating investigation, diagnosis and appropriate treatment.

Liver (vitamin A)

Although pregnant women do need small amounts of this vitamin, found in liver, it should not be consumed in large amounts or taken in dietary supplements as this may have teratogenic effects on the developing fetus. Vitamin A is also found in fish liver oils, therefore such supplements should be avoided in pregnancy (Food Standards Agency 2008a).

Vitamin D

It is recommended that women take vitamin D supplement of 10 μg of vitamin D each day during pregnancy (Rothman et al 1995, NICE 2008). Vitamin D helps regulate the amount of calcium and phosphate in the body, which are required for the formation of bones and teeth (Food Standards Agency 2008a).

Swordfish, marlin and shark

These fish should not be eaten due to their high methylmercury content, which could affect the nervous system of the developing fetus (Food Standards Agency 2008a). There is evidence to suggest that women who consume a low seafood diet are more at risk of premature labour (Olsen & Secher 2002) although further evidence is required from randomized controlled trials to support these findings. Professionals should always be aware of the impact of their advice. Enkin et al (2000:41) suggest caution and state:

efforts to encourage women to eat well during pregnancy, however well intentioned, often include explicit statements that women can reduce their risk of having a pre-term infant through attention to their diet and other lifestyle issues. Such statements are not only misleading, but can engender guilt, anxiety and a false sense of responsibility for untoward pregnancy outcomes.

Folic acid and iron

It is recommended that women have a diet rich in folic acid and take folic acid supplementation prior to conception and up to the 12th week of pregnancy, to reduce the risk of having a baby with a neural tube defect (Wald et al 1991). The recommended dose is 400 μg daily (NICE 2008). Folic acid is also important for the formation of red blood cells and folic acid rich foods include sprouts, asparagus, peas and broccoli, oranges and bananas (Food Standards Agency 2008a). Women should also ensure that their diet is rich in iron, which is necessary for the production of red blood cells. Iron rich foods include red meat, fortified cereals, grains and pulses and leafy green vegetables (Food Standards Agency 2008a). There is no evidence that routine iron supplementation has any benefit on the health outcomes of either mother or baby (Pena-Rosas & Viteri 2006) and they are not recommended as part of routine antenatal care (NICE 2008).

Box 4.1 lists changes occurring during pregnancy which have an effect on dietary intake.

Box 4.1: Changes during pregnancy impacting on dietary intake

■ **Nausea and vomiting**

Affects 70% of pregnant women, exacerbated by fatigue, some symptoms relieved by small, frequent, high carbohydrate meals. Acupressure is helpful for some women (Steele et al 2001). Most problematic during first trimester although persists throughout pregnancy in 20% of women (Coad et al 2000). There is some evidence that vitamin B6 may help reduce the severity of nausea (Jewell Young 1996).

■ **Increased appetite and thirst**

Experienced by more than 50% of women (Coad 2001). Capacity of the stomach reduced in late pregnancy due to displacement by gravid uterus.

■ **Cravings**

Women sometimes have cravings for unusual food combinations during pregnancy and these are usually harmless. Alternatively, women may develop a dislike for foods and drinks normally enjoyed, such as tea and coffee. This may be exacerbated by a metallic taste in the mouth. Consuming or craving substances that have no nutritional food value is known as 'pica'.

■ **Increased salivation**

The term 'ptyalism' refers to the experience of excess saliva in the mouth, although there is no evidence to confirm excess production but rather that swallowing saliva induces nausea in some women resulting in a tendency for it to collect in the mouth (Stables Rankin 2005).

■ **Indigestion**

Increased progesterone levels lead to impaired competence of the cardiac sphincter of the stomach. Reflux acid causes epigastric pain exacerbated by large or spicy meals. Maintaining an upright posture can help prevent gastric reflux. Antacids are sometimes required to alleviate symptoms, although long-term use may disrupt acid production (Jordan 2002).

continued

> **Box 4.1:** Continued
>
> ■ **Constipation**
>
> Relaxation of smooth muscle of gastrointestinal tract due to progesterone. Slower passage of food, increased absorption of water. Constipation may be exacerbated by some oral iron therapy. Need to increase fibre content of diet, e.g. cereals, fresh fruit and vegetables. A systematic review of interventions for treating constipation in pregnancy concluded that bowel stimulants were more effective than bulking agents but were more likely to lead to abdominal pain and diarrhoea (Jewell Young 1998). Haemorrhoids may compound the problem.

Activity

Find out what is meant by hyperemesis gravidarum.

See if you can discover what is the incidence and who is most at risk of this condition.

Find out how the midwife would recognize this condition, and what the treatment is.

Salt

A systematic review of the evidence related to reducing salt intake in pregnancy with a view to preventing or reducing the risk of pre-eclampsia did not show any evidence of benefit to mother or baby (Duley et al 2005). It is, however, a recommendation that adults do not consume more than 6 g of salt daily, to reduce the risk of hypertension and associated vascular disease (Food Standards Agency 2008b).

Caffeine

The Food Standards Agency (2008) recommends that women should not consume more than 300 mg of caffeine per day (3 mugs of coffee) as excessive intake has been linked to low birthweight and miscarriage. A study by Cnattingius et al (2000) found an increased risk of spontaneous abortion at levels of caffeine consumption above 100 mg. There are also other sources of caffeine that need to be taken into account (tea 50 mg, cola 40 mg, chocolate 50 mg and some cold remedies).

Lifestyle choices

Alcohol

Midwives need to find ways to explore women's alcohol consumption in a sensitive, non-judgmental way as it is thought that under reporting is widespread (RCOG 2006a). A consistently high consumption of alcohol is linked with a series of characteristics that together are known as fetal alcohol syndrome (FAS). They include mental retardation, microcephaly, small eyes, hearing disorders, large ears, shallow philtrum, small for gestational age, thin lips and congenital abnormalities (Seidel et al 1997). Binge drinking has been highlighted as being particularly harmful (RCOG 2006a). The Food Standards Agency recommend that women abstain from drinking alcohol throughout pregnancy, however, when women do continue to drink, consumption should not exceed one to two units once or twice a week (FSA 2008). A study (Kesmodel et al 2002) found an increasing risk of stillbirth with increasing moderate alcohol consumption.

Smoking

Both professionals and members of the public are well aware that smoking is hazardous to extra-uterine and intra-uterine health (Tobacco Information Campaign 2002). However, despite this knowledge, many pregnant women and their partners continue to smoke. They need support to give up and there are many local initiatives designed to provide advice and encouragement. Access to services depends on the midwife identifying the need for support and using her interpersonal skills to discuss the topic in a non-judgmental manner. The midwife needs to be aware of her own feelings with regard to women who smoke. If she alienates her when she asks the first question, 'Do you smoke?' either by the tone of her voice or the look on her face, it may be very difficult to repair the damage. It is important not to push information on a woman who does not want to give up smoking;

however, it is prudent to assess if the woman is aware of the dangers to both herself and the developing fetus, and to correct misinformation. Even if a woman does not choose to make changes based on the information she receives, she still has a right to informed choice about her health behaviour.

Activity

Consider the pregnant woman who, when asked by the midwife if she knows the risks of smoking in pregnancy replies, 'My friend had an 8 lb baby last week and she smoked all the way through her pregnancy.' Think about what you would say to her.

The consequences of maternal smoking on the baby continue to emerge. They include: low birthweight (Cnattingius & Haglund 1997), acute and chronic middle ear disease (Strachan & Cook 1998), respiratory illness (Fergusson et al 1980; Weitzman et al 1990), increased risk of sudden infant death syndrome (Haglund & Cnattingius 1990) and reduced breastmilk volume in the mother (Vaio et al 1991).

Interventions to help smokers quit

A systematic review concluded that smoking cessation programmes in pregnancy are effective in reducing the number of women who smoke and have a subsequent impact on low birthweight and pre-term birth (Lumley et al 2004). Owen (2000) describes an evaluation of a telephone helpline, supported by an information pack. Of those who called the helpline, 15.6% had stopped smoking at one year and of those who resumed smoking, 28% were smoking less than they had been initially. Products containing controlled amounts of nicotine are available over the counter in the form of chewing-gum, patches and lozenges. They were previously contraindicated during pregnancy and breastfeeding and not available on the NHS. However, the National Institute for Health and Clinical Excellence (NICE) has undertaken technical appraisal of the use of nicotine replacement therapy (NRT) and the drug Bupropion (amfebutamone) (NICE 2002). It concluded that NRT could be prescribed (free of charge) to pregnant women following discussion with an appropriate healthcare professional with careful consideration of the risks and benefits. Breastfeeding or pregnant women should NOT take Bupropion (p 7).

Activity

Find out what facilities are available to help pregnant smokers to quit both at your hospital trust and in primary care.

Investigate whether this service has been evaluated.

If so, record the success rate and note how it is measured.

Drug dependency

Pregnant drug users have a range of social, emotional and physical needs that require expert attention. This vulnerable group of women requires individualized care. The Confidential Enquiry into Maternal Deaths 1997–1999 (CEMD 2001) identified 11 deaths from accidental drug overdose. There were two deaths attributed to overdose of street drugs in the triennium 2003–2005, and 11% of all the women who died had a problem with substance abuse (Lewis 2007). There are many more women who do not die as a result of their drug dependency but who remain vulnerable because of their chaotic domestic circumstances. The babies of drug users are also at risk of a range of sequelae, depending on the type of drug and degree of abuse (Baston & Durward 2001).

Women can be referred to local drug dependency services for care and treatment. The benefits of other interventions need further evaluation. Care across the childbirth continuum needs to be carefully coordinated between the members of the multi-professional team. Non-attendance for antenatal care must be followed up (Lewis 2007). A systematic review to determine the effects of home visits during pregnancy and/or after birth for women with an alcohol or drug problem (Doggett et al 2005) did not find any health benefits associated with this intervention. There was evidence however that home visits after the birth did enhance women's engagement with drug treatment services.

Activity during pregnancy

Fatigue

People often associate fatigue in pregnancy with carrying an extra load around. Whilst this does contribute during the last trimester, it does not explain the debilitating lack of energy in the early weeks. Feeling tired in pregnancy can be extremely frustrating. Early pregnancy is particularly difficult as women have little to show in the way of a swelling abdomen, yet feel that they need to go to bed much earlier than usual. Women need reassurance that it is normal to feel very tired in the first trimester and that it will pass. Partners also need this information as reassurance that they will not spend every evening alone during the pregnancy. Providing feedback regarding the full blood count at booking is useful, women may fear that they are anaemic and this needs to be ruled out or treated.

Activity

Check that you know what the midwife is looking for when she looks at a full blood count result.

Make sure you understand why some women experience dizziness or fainting when pregnant.

Think about what advice the midwife can offer.

Exercise

Moderate exercise during a low-risk pregnancy has not been shown to put the fetus or mother at risk. It has the advantage of maintaining flexibility, enhancing self-esteem and has beneficial cardiac and respiratory effects. The Royal College of Obstetricians and Gynaecologists recommend that all women should be encouraged to 'participate in aerobic and strength conditioning exercise as part of a healthy lifestyle during their pregnancy' (RCOG 2006b:01). Contact sports should, however, be avoided, along with those that put excessive stress on the joints, which are more mobile in pregnancy. Women should take measures to avoid over-heating during exercise and ensure that they reduce the risk of hypoglycaemia by limiting exercise sessions to no more than 45 minutes and consuming sufficient calories (Soultanakis et al 1996). Pregnant women should also avoid exercising in the supine position as this may lead to vena caval compression.

A small study by Bungum et al (2000) concluded that exercise may contribute to a reduced risk of caesarean section. Women who did not previously exercise should be advised to start with non-weightbearing exercise, such as swimming. Regular, moderate exercise is better than sporadic, strenuous exertion and women should still be able to talk during exercise. Sexual activity during pregnancy, for women with an uncomplicated pregnancy, is not associated with adverse outcomes.

Indeed a recent study (Sayle et al 2001) concluded that intercourse during late pregnancy was associated with a reduced risk of pre-term delivery.

Symphysis pubis dysfunction

Activity may be severely restricted if the woman develops a condition known as symphysis pubis dysfunction (SPD). The effect of the hormone relaxin leads to separation of the symphysis pubis, which in extreme cases makes weightbearing impossible (Wellock 2002). Women who develop this painful condition need a lot of support and individualized care. They should be referred to an obstetric physiotherapist for specialist advice. Treatment is rest and the condition may persist for several months following the birth.

Backache

Backache affects 48–90% of pregnant woman (Lennard 2002). A combination of increased progesterone and relaxin circulation, increased weight gain and altered posture contribute to pain that can be mild to severe, constant or intermittent. Interventions that have been demonstrated to be helpful include aquarobics, physiotherapy and acupuncture (Young & Jewell 2002), and specifically tailored strengthening and stretching exercises (Pennick & Young 1998).

Rest during pregnancy

Although moderate exercise is beneficial during pregnancy, a balance between activity and rest that meets the individual woman's requirement is important. There is no evidence that rest should be forced upon women, for example, to reduce the risk of miscarriage (Aleman et al 2005).

Unfortunately, many women experience difficulties maintaining their pre-pregnancy sleeping patterns and this can be a source of anxiety. Pregnant women may experience disturbed sleep patterns for many reasons (Mindell & Jacobson 2000). The midwife needs to carefully explore a range of issues with women who complain of lack of or disturbed sleep in order to give appropriate advice. Ultimately, the woman may need to alter her usual sleep and rest patterns during her pregnancy.

Uncomfortable in bed

Women who had previously slept on their front may soon find that this position is no longer possible, due to an enlarging abdomen and/or breast tenderness. It can be helpful not only to suggest, but also to demonstrate how a pillow under the abdomen and one in between the legs can help a woman sleep comfortably on her side. It is not advisable for pregnant women to sleep on their back as the weight of the gravid uterus on the vena cava can impede venous return causing a drop in blood pressure and oxygen supply to the fetus. Women are also more likely to snore in pregnancy, following changes in nasal mucosa (Santiago et al 2001) and snoring is also exacerbated by sleeping on the back, further disturbing the pattern of sleep.

Fetal movements at night

Women tend to notice the baby's movements more during a rest period because their work or general activities do not distract them. Also, the baby seems to enjoy the increased blood flow and oxygen supply, as they are not competing with active muscles. Fetal movements are a sign of wellbeing and should be enjoyed; however, the woman may need help to relax in spite of her active baby. Simple relaxation techniques can be practised and a warm bath before bedtime may help as the baby can have its active period then, instead of when she gets into bed.

Cramp

Cramp of the legs can be severe, bringing an abrupt end to a deep sleep. Exercising the muscles before bedtime, by rapid and repeated flexion and extension of each foot, can help disperse the build-up of lactic acid that causes the pain. During an acute attack of cramp, the offending foot should be pulled towards the body, to extend the calf muscle (easier said than done when heavily pregnant). Alternatively, the foot can be pressed against the wall or standing up with the leg behind the body (but this involves getting out of bed). A systematic review of interventions for leg cramps in pregnancy concluded that where this is a persistent problem, magnesium lactate or citrate 5 mmol in the morning and 10 mmol in the evening is the most appropriate treatment (Young & Jewell 1996).

Frequency of micturition

This is a problem particularly in the first and third trimesters of pregnancy. In the first trimester the growing uterus is a pelvic organ and shares the space with the bladder. Women need to be reassured that this problem will pass (albeit to return later) and it is useful to show a picture demonstrating the position of the pelvic and abdominal contents in relation to one another, to help her appreciate how her body is changing. In the last few weeks of pregnancy, as the presenting part enters the pelvis, there is the same competition for space. However, there is the additional factor that the baby can move its head or bottom, and exert pressure on the already compromised bladder, resulting in an urgent need for the woman to pass urine. Some might argue that the need to get up out of a lovely cosy bed, at repeated intervals during the night, is nature's way of preparing the woman for the joys of motherhood. On the other hand, the woman probably feels that she would rather prepare for the joys ahead by getting some good quality sleep. I remember the advice my colleague gave to the partners of women approaching this aspect of their pregnancy: 'speak kindly to her and put the covers back to keep the bed warm for her return.'

Carpal tunnel syndrome

This condition is not exclusive to pregnancy, but can arise during pregnancy in women who have not experienced it at other times. It is caused by swelling or compression in the space in the wrist where the nerve travels to the hand. It results in pain and/or paraesthesia in the hand, which then leads the woman to wake up. She may not realize at first what is waking her up. Elevating the arm on a pillow or the use of a splint may provide some relief, but the condition may not resolve until after the birth.

Aching legs

Progesterone relaxes vascular tone, making the valves in the veins less effective and impeding venous return. Compounded by the pressure exerted by the gravid uterus, development of varicose veins in the legs and perineal region can be problematic. In addition, uncomfortable, fidgety legs are often an irritation during pregnancy. Gentle exercise, such as ankle rotation, can provide temporary relief. The woman can be advised to elevate her legs while sitting, if possible. Support tights may also help and prevent or reduce the risk of oedema.

Activity

Find out whether oedema is normal during pregnancy.

Make sure you know how and when the midwife should assess the woman for the development of varicose veins.

Make sure you can explain why varicose veins need to be observed.

Think about what advice the midwife can offer on this subject.

Find out what treatment is recommended in your locality.

Reflection on trigger scenario

Look back on the trigger scenario.

Joanna is now 20 weeks pregnant. She has been well, although rather nauseous at times, but this is now less frequent. She gave up smoking 3 weeks ago and is now beginning to struggle. She even got to the stage where she took one of Louis's cigarettes from the packet and searched through the kitchen drawer to find a lighter that worked. She was interrupted by an interesting text message and then managed to gather her willpower to put the cigarette back in its packet.

The scenario highlights how addressing a health behaviour, such as smoking, can be challenging and difficult to manage alone. It also emphasizes the need to engage women's partners in the experience of pregnancy, so that they can provide support and prepare for their new role. Now that you are familiar with the issues in relation to health in pregnancy, you should have insight into how the scenario relates to the evidence. The jigsaw model will now be used to explore the trigger scenario in more depth.

Effective communication

Joanna has decided to give up smoking and this is going well so far. However, she has found that she is filling the time she would usually be spending smoking with eating and this has led to a significant weight gain in a relatively short period of time.

Questions that arise from the scenario might include: How has Joanna received the message that she should give up smoking during pregnancy? Has it come from a health professional or through the media, family or peer group? What is the most effective method of changing health behaviours? How are women encouraged to access information about healthy lifestyles where you work?

Woman-centred care

Information about health in pregnancy should be specific to the individual needs of the woman. Questions that arise from the scenario might include: Did Joanna receive tailored information about her smoking habit at the booking history? Was the information given relevant and applicable to her current circumstances? Were her questions answered and any need for referral followed up? Was Joanna given information about local services that could help her address her smoking habit? Was an individual plan developed and documented with a plan for review discussed? How was Louis included in Joanna's plans to quit smoking?

Using best evidence

There are many interventions available to help women stop smoking, some specifically for those who are pregnant. Questions that arise from the scenario might include: Were different options for support to stop smoking discussed with Joanna? How are midwives informed of the most effective methods available? Are there evidence-based

programmes of care available in your locality? Is there an evidence-based policy or pathway available for use when a pregnant woman books for maternity care? Do you know how many pregnant smokers attempt to stop smoking and succeed? Is there an on-going audit of local smoking cessation programmes? What do the NICE guidelines recommend about smoking in pregnancy?

Professional and legal issues

It is part of the midwife's role to offer advice in pregnancy and to counsel women about their health behaviours (ICM 2005). Questions that arise from the scenario might include: How do midwives keep up-to-date with new evidence about health in pregnancy? Are workshops/information sessions provided at the Trust where you work? How can you identify and address your learning needs? What might be the potential consequences if you did not inform a woman about the risks she was taking by continuing to smoke during pregnancy? How do you document the advice you have given to women?

Team working

The midwife works as part of a team of professionals, each with an area of expertise and experience. Questions that arise from the scenario might include: Which professionals will Joanna already have come into contact with by this stage of her pregnancy? Which professionals would be best placed to discuss smoking cessation? Is there someone in your locality with a specific role in supporting pregnant women to stop smoking? What do you do when an issue is outside your area of expertise? How do you communicate with other members of the healthcare team?

Clinical dexterity

The midwife who refers a woman for help with smoking cessation will need an understanding of the techniques that are used to support this process even if she does not use them herself. The most important clinical skill will be sensitive interview techniques to gather accurate information and provide genuine emotional support. Questions that arise from the scenario might include: What interventions are used in your locality to support pregnant women who smoke? What do nicotine patches look like and how are they applied? How much nicotine do the patches prescribed in pregnancy contain? Are patches worn all day? Are other methods used to monitor compliance, such as nicotine breath detectors?

Models of care

The model of care that the woman is following could have significant implications for her success in making a change to her smoking status. This applies not only to the model of maternity care, for example, if she is receiving continuous support from a midwife, but also with regard to the smoking cessation programme she is following. Questions that arise from

the scenario might include: Does the antenatal documentation enable all professionals involved in care to follow Joanna's progress? Is Joanna supported on a one-to-one basis or is there a local group for peer support? Are there processes in place to enable Joanna to seek advice and support in between appointments?

Safe environment

The midwife needs to ensure that she provides a safe environment for women to disclose their individual circumstances so that appropriate individualized care can be offered. She also needs to monitor that prescribed treatments or interventions are being used appropriately. Questions that arise from the scenario might include: Is there sufficient privacy and time within the provision of antenatal care to enable women to disclose their concerns? How can the current system/environment be adapted to enhance communication? What is the regime for smoking cessation intervention locally?

Promotes health

The midwife has many opportunities throughout the antenatal period to promote the current and future health of women and their families. Questions that arise from the scenario might include: If Joanna quits smoking in pregnancy, how can she be supported to continue her abstinence once the baby is born? How can the midwife use this opportunity to promote the health of the baby? What information can the midwife give Joanna that will help her confront members of the family who smoke and prepare them to maintain a smoke-free environment for the new baby?

Further scenarios

The following scenarios enable you to consider how specific situations influence the care the midwife provides. Use the jigsaw model to explore the issues raised in the scenario.

Scenario 1

Lisa has given up smoking but she has become rather fond of the pastries on sale at the shop near her work. She is 22 weeks' pregnant and has already put on over a stone in weight.

Practice point

Further questions specific to Scenario 1 include:

1. Was Lisa warned that stopping smoking might initially lead to a gain in weight?
2. What strategies can the midwife suggest to help Lisa from putting on unnecessary weight?
3. NICE guidance states that repeated weighing during pregnancy should only be undertaken if it might influence clinical management (NICE 2008:23). How might this be interpreted?

4. Which other members of the healthcare team could potentially support Lisa to eat a balanced diet?

Scenario 2

Lucy has just found out she is 6 weeks pregnant. She is a keen horse rider and is about to take part in a national competition. She contacts her local community midwife for advice about continuing with this sport.

Practice point

Further questions specific to Scenario 2 include:

1. What does the evidence say about horse riding in pregnancy?
2. What other sources of information are available to women?
3. What are the potential risks and benefits of Lucy continuing to ride while pregnant?
4. What are your own personal feelings about competitive sports and pregnancy?
5. What is your role as a midwife in relation to giving advice?

Conclusion

Pregnancy makes many emotional and physical demands on the woman. She will value the support and experience of the midwives who care for her as she faces new challenges and makes choices about her lifestyle. The midwife has an important public health role that reaches beyond the childbirth continuum.

Resources

Adult obesity care pathway: www.dh.gov.uk/prod_consum_dh/idcplg?IdcService=GET_FILE&dID=24676&Rendition=Web.

Department of Health: http://www.dh.gov.uk/en/index.htm.

Food Standards Agency: http://www.eatwell.gov.uk/agesandstages/pregnancy/whenyrpregnant/.

Healthy Start: http://www.healthystart.nhs.uk/.

National Insitute for Health and Clinical Excellence: http://www.nice.org.uk/.

NHS Direct: http://www.nhsdirect.nhs.uk/.

Quit smoking on the NHS: http://gosmokefree.nhs.uk/?WT.mc_id=ilevel_search_08.

References

Aleman A, Althabe F, Belizan J, et al: Bed rest during pregnancy for preventing miscarriage, *Cochrane Database of Systematic Reviews* 2(CD003576), 2005.

Barker D: The fetal and infant origins of adult disease, *British Medical Journal* 301:1111, 1992.

Baston H, Durward H: *Examination of the newborn*, London, 2001, Routledge.

Bungum TJ, Peaslee DL, Jackson AW, et al: Exercise during pregnancy and type of delivery in nulliparae, *Journal of Obstetric, Gynaecologic and Neonatal Nursing* 29(3):258–264, 2000.

CEMD: *Why mothers die 1997–1999. The fifth report of the confidential enquiry into maternal deaths in the United Kingdom*, London, 2001, RCOG.

Claesson I, Sydsjo G, Brynhildsen J, et al: Weight gain restriction for obese pregnant women: a case control intervention study, *BJOG: an International Journal of Obstetrics & Gynaecology* 115(1):44–50, 2008.

Cnattingius S, Haglund B: Decreasing smoking prevalence during pregnancy in Sweden: the effect on small-for-gestational-age births, *American Journal of Public Health* 87(3):410–413, 1997.

Cnattingius S, Signorello LB, Anneren G, et al: Caffeine intake and the risk of first trimester spontaneous abortion, *New England Journal of Medicine* 343(25):1839–1845, 2000.

Coad J: *Anatomy and physiology for midwives*, Edinburgh, 2001, Mosby.

Coad J, Al-Rasasi B, Morgan J: New insights into nausea and vomiting in pregnancy, *MIDIRS Midwifery Digest* 10(4):451–454, 2000.

Department of Health: *Healthy Start: Reform of the Welfare Food Scheme*, London, 2004, Department of Health.

Doggett C, Burrett S, Osborn DA: Home visits during pregnancy and after birth for women with an alcohol or drug problem, *Cochrane Database of Systematic Reviews* 4(CD004456), 2005.

Duley L, Henderson-Smart D, Meher S: Altered dietary salt for preventing pre-eclampsia, and its complications, *Cochrane Database of Systematic Reviews* 4(CD005548), 2005.

Enkin M, Keirse MJNC, Neilson J, et al: *A guide to effective care in pregnancy and childbirth*, ed 3, Oxford, 2000, Oxford University Press.

Fergusson DM, Horwood LJ, Shannon FT: Parental smoking and respiratory illness in infancy, *Archives of Disease in Childhood* 55(5):358–361, 1980.

Food Standards Agency: Eat well, be well, 2008a. Online. Available http://www.eatwell.gov.uk/healthydiet/nutritionessentials/vitaminsandminerals/ April 29, 2008.

Food Standards Agency, 2008b. Online. Available http://www.food.gov.uk/healthiereating/salt/ April 19, 2008.

Frohlich J: Obesity in pregnancy, *MIDIRS Midwifery Digest* 12(1):39–43, 2002.

Haglund B, Cnattingius S: Cigarette smoking as a risk factor for sudden infant death syndrome: a population-based study, *American Journal of Public Health* 80(1):29–32, 1990.

International Confederation of Midwives: Definition of a midwife, 2005. Online. Available http://www.medicalknowledgeinstitute.com/files/ICM%20Definition%20of%20the%20Midwife%202005.pdf April 29, 2008.

Jewell D, Young G: Interventions for nausea and vomiting in early pregnancy, *Cochrane Database of Systematic Reviews* 4(CD000145), 1996.

Jewell D, Young D: Interventions for treating constipation in pregnancy, *Cochrane Database of Systematic Reviews* 3(CD001142), 1998.

Jordan S: *Pharmacology for midwives: the evidence base for safe practice*, Basingstoke, 2002, Palgrave.

Kesmodel U, Wisborg K, Olsen SF, et al: Moderate alcohol intake during pregnancy and the risk of still birth and death in the first year of life, *American Journal of Epidemiology* 155(4):305–312, 2002.

Kramer MS: Balanced protein/energy supplementation in pregnancy. *Cochrane Review. Cochrane Library*, Issue 3. Oxford, 2008, Update Software.

Lennard F: An introduction to back and pelvic pain during pregnancy, *British Journal of Midwifery* 10(12):736–740, 2002.

Lewis G, editor: *Confidential enquiry into maternal and child health. Improving the health of mothers, babies and children. Why mothers die 2000–2002. Midwifery summary and key recommendations*, London, 2004, RCOG.

Lewis G, editor: *The confidential enquiry into maternal and child health (CEMACH). Saving mothers' lives: reviewing maternal deaths to make motherhood safer – 2003–2005. The seventh report on confidential enquiries into maternal deaths in the United Kingdom*, London, 2007, CEMACH.

Lumley J, Oliver S, Chaberlain C, et al: Intervention for promoting smoking cessation during pregnancy, *Cochrane Database of Systematic Reviews* 4(CD001055), 2004.

Mindell JA, Jacobson BJ: Sleep disturbances during pregnancy, *Journal of Obstetric, Gynaecological and Neonatal Nursing* 29(6):590–597, 2000.

National Institute for Health and Clinical Excellence (NICE): *Guidance on the use of nicotine replacement therapy and Bupropion for smoking cessation: Technology Guidance No 39*, London, 2002, NICE.

National Institute for Health and Clinical Excellence (NICE): *Antenatal care: routine care for the healthy pregnant woman. Clinical guideline 62*, London, 2008, National Collaborating Centre for Women's and Children's Health.

Olsen SF, Secher NJ: Low consumption of seafood in early pregnancy as a factor for preterm delivery: a prospective cohort study, *British Medical Journal* 324(7335):447–450, 2002.

Owen L: Impact of a telephone helpline for smokers who called during a mass media campaign, *Tobacco Control* 9:148–154, 2000.

Pena-Rosas J, Viteri F: Effects of routine oral iron supplementation with or without folic acid for women during pregnancy, *Cochrane Database of Systematic Reviews* 3(CD004736), 2006.

Pennick V, Young G: Interventions for preventing and treating pelvic and back pain in pregnancy, *Cochrane Database of Systematic Reviews* 3(CD001139), 1998.

Richens Y: Tackling maternal obesity: suggestions for midwives, *British Journal of Midwifery* 16(1):14–18, 2008.

Rothman KJ, Moore LL, Singer MR, et al: Teratogenicity of high vitamin A intake, *New England Journal of Medicine* 333(21):1369–1373, 1995.

Royal College of Obstetricians and Gynaecologists (RCOG): Alcohol consumption and the outcomes of pregnancy. Statement No 5, 2006a. Online. Available http://www.rcog.org.uk/resources/Public/pdf/alcohol_pregnancy_rcog_statement5a.pdf April 20, 2008.

Royal College of Obstetricians and Gynaecologists (RCOG): Exercise in pregnancy. Statement No 4, 2006b. Online. Available http://www.rcog.org.uk/resources/Public/pdf/exercise_pregnancy_rcog_statement4.pdf April 20, 2008.

Royal College of Obstetricians and Gynaecologists: Obesity and reproductive health, 2007. Online. Available http://www.rcog.org.uk/resources/public/pdf/study_gp_obesity.pdf April 19, 2008.

Santiago JR, Nolledo MS, Kinzler W, et al: Sleep and sleep disorders in pregnancy, *Annals of Internal Medicine* 134(5):396–408, 2001.

Sayle AE, Savitz DA, Thorp JM, et al: Sexual activity during late pregnancy and risk of preterm delivery, *Obstetrics and Gynecology* 97(2):283–289, 2001.

Seidel HM, Rosenstein BJ, Pathak A: *Primary care of the newborn*, ed 2, St Louis, 1997, Mosby.

Soultanakis H, Artal R, Wisewell R: Prolonged exercise in pregnancy: glucose homeostasis, ventilatory and cardiovascular responses, *Seminars in Perinatology* 20(4):315–327, 1996.

Stables D, Rankin J: *Physiology in childbearing with anatomy and related biosciences*, Edinburgh, 2005, Elsevier.

Steele NM, French J, Gatherer-Boyle, et al: Effect of acupressure by sea-bands on nausea and vomiting of pregnancy. *Journal of Gynecologic and Neonatal Nursing* 30(1):61–70, 2001.

Strachan DP, Cook DG: Health effects of passive smoking. 4: Parental smoking, middle ear disease and adenotonsillectomy in children, *Thorax* 53(1):50–56, 1998.

Tieu J, Crowther C, Middleton P: Dietary advice in pregnancy for preventing gestational diabetes mellitus, *Cochrane Database of Systematic Reviews* 2(CD006674), 2008.

Tobacco Information Campaign: Helping pregnant women to stop smoking, *British Journal of Midwifery* 10(11):663–667, 2002.

Vaio F, Salazar G, Infante C: Smoking during pregnancy and lactation and its effects on breast-milk volume, *American Journal of Nutrition* 54(6):1011–1016, 1991.

Wald N, Sneddon J, Densem J, et al: Prevention of neural tube defects: Results of the medical research council vitamin study, *The Lancet* 338(8760):131–137, 1991.

Watkins M, Ramussen S, Honein M, et al: Maternal obesity and risk for birth defects, *Pediatrics* 111(5):1132–1158, 2003.

Wellock V: The ever widening gap: symphysis pubis dysfunction, *British Journal of Midwifery* 10(6):348–353, 2002.

Weitzman M, Gorunaker S, Walker DK, et al: Maternal smoking and childhood asthma, *Pediatrics* 85(4):505–511, 1990.

Young G, Jewell D: Interventions for leg cramps in pregnancy, *Cochrane Database of Systematic Reviews* 2(CD000121), 1996.

Young G, Jewell D: Interventions for preventing and treating pelvic and back pain in pregnancy, *Cochrane Database of Systematic Reviews*, 1(CD000121), 2002.

Chapter 5

Monitoring maternal physical wellbeing

Trigger scenario

Joanna is now 25 weeks pregnant. She has just returned from her antenatal check-up with the midwife. It was not the same midwife who had taken her booking history but she was friendly and took time to read through Jo's records. The midwife said that her blood pressure was up a bit, but when she retook it later it was fine. Jo had meant to ask her midwife what she should take for heartburn, but did not get the chance. She will call in at the chemist on her way to work.

Introduction

This chapter focuses on aspects of the 'antenatal check' undertaken by the midwife that monitor the physical wellbeing of the pregnant woman. Previous chapters have examined the procedure and rationale for some of the clinical activities undertaken by the midwife to assess the woman's health status. During assessment of maternal physical health, the midwife will undertake an evaluation of her emotional wellbeing, and issues surrounding this aspect of care will be considered in further detail in the following chapter. Aspects of the examination that address assessment of fetal wellbeing, including abdominal palpation, will be discussed in Chapter 9.

The antenatal check

The National Institute for Health and Clinical Excellence has published recommendations regarding the content and frequency of antenatal appointments (NICE 2008) and these are summarized in Table 5.1. It is recommended that, following their initial contact with a health professional to confirm pregnancy, nulliparous women should have 10 antenatal appointments and multiparous women should have seven (NICE 2008:50). A large national survey of women's experience of maternity care (Redshaw et al 2006) reported that there was little difference between the number of antenatal checks for women who had babies before, with an overall average of 10 checks.

The midwife should be mindful that the NICE Antenatal care guideline is a guideline for 'healthy pregnant women' and where women need more support or additional monitoring this should be scheduled accordingly. Ultimately care should be tailored to meet the needs of individual women. For example: a woman experiencing a normal second pregnancy may not need to be seen as often as a woman who has a history of infertility. However, this assumption is based on generalization. The woman expecting her second baby may have had a traumatic first birth or a sister who has had a stillbirth. She may require a lot of additional support from the professional she meets. The woman with a history of infertility may be happy and well, and content to be seen according to the usual schedule. One of the many benefits of continuity of antenatal care is that the midwife can establish and maintain relationships with women, noticing when circumstances change and when the way care is offered needs to adapt in response.

Record keeping

Throughout midwifery practice, our records facilitate effective care and can be used to repeat and confirm our assessment and plan of action with the woman. She should be shown what is written, so that it can be explained there and then, rather than her going away and wondering what it all means. At the end of the interaction, the woman should understand the implications of any findings and what happens next. Finally, she should be invited to ask any more questions.

Table 5.1 shows a schedule of antenatal appointments for primiparous and multiparous women, together with the content of the visits.

Safety

The woman attending for her antenatal check-up has probably been anticipating it (either with joy or dread) for several days beforehand. She may have thought of questions she wanted to ask or have been worried that her blood pressure might be up again. In an exploratory study, Melender & Lauri (2001) linked women's sense of security in pregnancy with visits to the clinic, good relationships with the midwife, and screening tests. The challenge for the midwife with many women to see in a busy antenatal clinic is to enable each woman to feel that she has been treated with respect and as an individual. Staff shortages, study leave and sickness compound to make this a tall order. However, eye contact, acknowledgement and active listening will enhance the interaction, without substantially lengthening the consultation. When a woman obviously needs more time, depending on the structure of local services and her current health status, it may be possible to offer a home visit or schedule another appointment.

Table 5.1 Schedule of antenatal appointments and content

When	Primparous	Multiparous
First contact with a health professional: confirmation of pregnancy		
Booking (by 10 weeks)	Blood tests for blood group, rhesus factor, anaemia, haemoglobinopathies, red-cell alloantibodies, hepatitis B virus, HIV, rubella antibodies and syphylis Offer dating and anomaly scans and information on antenatal screening tests	Blood tests for blood group, rhesus factor, anaemia, haemoglobinopathies, red-cell alloantibodies, hepatitis B virus, HIV, rubella antibodies and syphylis Offer dating and anomaly scans and information on antenatal screening tests
16 weeks	Blood pressure and urinalysis Review screening tests Information giving	Blood pressure and urinalysis Review screening tests Information giving
25 weeks	Blood pressure and urinalysis Information giving Symphysis–fundal height	
28 weeks	Blood pressure and urinalysis Information giving Symphysis–fundal height Offer anti-D prophylaxis to rhesus negative women Screen for anaemia and atypical red-cell alloantibodies	Blood pressure and urinalysis Information giving Symphysis–fundal height Offer anti-D prophylaxis to rhesus negative women Screen for anaemia and atypical red-cell alloantibodies
31 weeks	Blood pressure and urinalysis Information giving Symphysis–fundal height Review screening	
34 weeks	Blood pressure and urinalysis Information giving Symphysis–fundal height Offer 2nd anti-D prophylaxis to rhesus negative women	Blood pressure and urinalysis Information giving Symphysis–fundal height Offer 2nd anti-D prophylaxis to rhesus negative women
36 weeks	Blood pressure and urinalysis Information giving Symphysis–fundal height Check position of baby	Blood pressure and urinalysis Information giving Symphysis–fundal height Check position of baby

Continued

Table 5.1 Continued

When	Primparous	Multiparous
38 weeks	Blood pressure and urinalysis Information giving	Blood pressure and urinalysis Information giving
40 weeks	Blood pressure and urinalysis Information giving	
41 weeks	Blood pressure and urinalysis Information giving Offer a membrane sweep Offer induction of labour	Blood pressure and urinalysis Information giving Offer a membrane sweep Offer induction of labour

The woman must feel that the room is safe, that the door will not suddenly be opened and a private conversation or disclosure interrupted. She also needs to feel that the information she offers will not be passed around the staff room or to the next woman in the waiting room. She will judge this by the midwife's interactions with her. For example, if the midwife is not telling her about the previous person or the woman who lives next door, then this will give her more confidence that the midwife will not discuss her circumstances with others either.

Emotional wellbeing

The emotions that women experience during their pregnancy are wide ranging. They may change over the duration of the pregnancy and differ between individual pregnancies. The woman may need to explore her feelings with a midwife and an opening question, such as 'How are you feeling?', provides such an opportunity. Emotional support is identified by Wheatley (1998:46–47) as:

all those instances where reassurance, intimacy and the knowledge that one is loved and cared for are received, when advice is either sought from or offered by someone who can be confided in and relied upon to help.

The mind and body are inextricably linked such that physical pathology may lead to emotional distress and vice versa. The midwife also needs to recognize the impact of maternal ill health on the wellbeing of the developing baby and conversely, that concern about the baby will affect the emotional health of the woman. The woman's general activity level and sprightliness may speak volumes, not just about her physical health, but also regarding her emotional health. It is good practice to go out to the waiting room and call the woman in personally. Doing so enables the midwife to assess her mobility and her mood. We can all put on a smile but much more than that is difficult to maintain if we are feeling low. Our body gives us away by our posture and eye contact.

Activity

Identify an example of how the discovery of physical illness in the mother could lead to her emotional distress. How would you minimize its effect?

Find out what services are available in your locality for pregnant women with mental health problems.

Social activity

Showing interest in the woman, rather than just the progress of the pregnancy, demonstrates concern for her as an individual. Knowledge of what the woman is doing will also provide insight into how she is feeling. It would be inappropriate to bombard the woman with a list of probing questions, but the midwife will need to satisfy herself that she is aware of the woman's social circumstances, particularly if she did not do the booking history at the woman's home. Is she getting support from her partner and are they making preparations together? Does she have family and friends in the area or is the woman socially isolated?

It is also important to follow up on issues that were highlighted during the booking history. For example, if the woman smoked and showed an interest in cutting down, it is important to find

out how her plans are going. She may have initially declined referral to a local support initiative, but now feels that she would like to take up the offer. If she is managing to cut down using her own willpower, support and encouragement may help her maintain her resolve.

Physical tests

Routine urinalysis

It is recommended that the woman's urine is tested for proteinuria at each antenatal examination (NICE 2008). She is asked to provide a midstream specimen in a clean container. Although a washed out jar or bottle will suffice, a specimen bottle is more discrete and secure, and can be washed and reused throughout the pregnancy. Proteinuria is an ominous symptom of pre-eclampsia; hypertensive disease in pregnancy is the second leading cause of maternal death in this country (Lewis et al 2007). There should not be any protein in urine; however, detection of a trace of protein may be present through contamination, and does not require further action unless associated with other signs of pathology.

Activity

Think about how you might discuss the finding of proteinuria with a woman. Work out how you might explain the significance, without alarming her. Make sure you know what further tests or follow-up might be indicated.

Box 5.1 Monitoring maternal wellbeing during pregnancy

• **INQUIRE ABOUT MOOD**

Rationale To identify women in need of additional support or specialist input. Take action if: feelings of hopelessness, self-harm, tocophobia, agitation, anxiety, obsessive thoughts

• **INQUIRE ABOUT GENERAL ACTIVITY**

Rationale To identify women with depressed mood, debilitating fatigue or physical pain in need of further investigation. Take action if: agoraphobia, inertia, extreme lethargy, pelvic pain

• **INQUIRE ABOUT SLEEP PATTERNS**

Rationale To identify poor quality/ quantity of sleep and offer advice. Take action if: insomnia, narcosis

• **BLOOD PRESSURE MEASUREMENT**

Rationale To confirm that blood pressure remains within safe parameters. Opportunity to give advice regarding action to take if signs or symptoms of pre-eclampsia arise. Take action if: systolic pressure above 140 mmHg and/or diastolic pressure above 90 mmHg, proteinurea, headaches, epigastric pain, visual disturbances

• **URINALYSIS**

Rationale To exclude the presence of protein. To detect infection or pre-eclampsia. Opportunity to give advice regarding action to take if signs or symptoms arise. Take action if: proteinurea, haematurea

• **LEG EXAMINATION**

Rationale To identify varicose veins or deep vein thrombosis. To monitor and advise regarding oedema. Opportunity to offer advice and referral if necessary. Take action if: different sized calves, hot, red areas, painful or swollen veins

• **BLOOD TESTS**

Rationale To detect and treat anaemia. To detect development of rhesus antibodies. Take action if: results outside normal parameters, depending on local policy

• **INQUIRE ABOUT ANY VAGINAL LOSS**

Rationale To detect possible infection, premature rupture of fetal membranes or placental separation. Opportunity to give advice regarding action to take if signs or symptoms arise. Take action if: blood loss, loss of liquor, offensive, itchy or discolored vaginal discharge

• **INQUIRE ABOUT BOWEL FUNCTION**

Rationale To identify need for dietary advice or side effects from iron therapy. Opportunity to offer preventative advice. Take action if: constipation, diarrhoea, haemorrhoids

• **INQUIRE ABOUT BLADDER FUNCTION**

Rationale To detect infection and offer advice regarding pelvic floor exercises. Takew action if: dysurea, incontinence

• **INQUIRE ABOUT DIETARY INTAKE**

Rationale To identify women with eating disorders, nausea and vomiting, poor nutrition or depression. Opportunity to offer advice. Take action if: bulimia, anorexia, malnutrition

Blood pressure measurement

Blood pressure is measured at each antenatal examination (NICE 2008). Women whose blood pressure falls outside the normal range (usually that which is greater than 140 mmHg systolic and/or 90 mmHg diastolic) should be followed up. Depending on the circumstances and local policy, the woman may be referred to an antenatal assessment unit for further monitoring. In the absence of proteinurea, other symptoms and a relatively small increase from the booking blood pressure reading, the midwife may arrange to repeat the blood pressure measurement in the woman's own home. Women should be informed to contact the hospital if they experience visual disturbances, severe headache or epigastric pain; there is a reminder on the National Maternity Records. However, many women with pre-eclampsia feel well. For detailed instruction how to take an accurate blood pressure, see Baston et al (2009) *Midwifery Essentials: Basics.*

Activity

Find out about Korotkoff sounds. Make sure you know which you should record during pregnancy.

Think of five questions you might ask the woman if her blood pressure is raised.

Blood tests

The booking blood results should be available and documented in the woman's maternity records by the 16-week appointment (NICE 2008). The woman should be informed of all results and their meaning should be explained. Abnormal results should be discussed with the woman and a clear plan of action documented. See Chapter 7 for further details regarding blood tests in pregnancy.

Clinical examination and inquiry

Legs

Thromboembolism is the leading cause of maternal death in the United Kingdom (Lewis 2007). The midwife should ask the woman if she has any pain in her legs and assess them by looking to see that they are both the same size (different sizes might occur if there is a deep vein thrombosis in the calf – measure them if there is any uncertainty). Uncomfortable varicose veins might benefit from support tights, but need careful monitoring for the development of phlebitis.

Tight, shiny skin may be present if the woman has marked oedema. If present, the midwife assesses the severity by asking how far up the leg it goes and gently depressing the skin in front of the tibia, to see if the skin remains depressed when the finger is removed. The further up the leg the indentation can be made, the more severe the oedema. The midwife should also ask if the oedema goes down at night, which it should. The hands and face should also be assessed. Although oedema is both common and normal in pregnancy, it can be associated with pre-eclampsia and should alert the midwife to exclude the development of this condition. Also, common or not, it is still uncomfortable and does not enhance the body image. The midwife can offer simple advice, regarding elevating legs when seated and regular leg exercises to improve venous return, but most importantly she should provide reassurance and understanding.

Vaginal loss

Any report of vaginal loss of fluid needs careful investigation. Bleeding in pregnancy is abnormal and necessitates further investigation to identify the cause. Women need to know the difference between a 'show' and antepartum haemorrhage. A 'show' is always mixed with mucus. Blood that soaks through the pants or runs down the leg requires prompt admission to the delivery suite. Watery vaginal loss also needs careful assessment. Liquor has a distinct smell and is clear or may be stained with meconium. It can be distinguished from urine, which is yellow. Women should be advised to wear a sanitary towel if they experience any vaginal loss so that it can be closely observed, and to speak to a midwife for advice.

It is normal for women to have a white vaginal discharge (leucorrhoea) during pregnancy that is heavier than when not pregnant. However, it should not be coloured, offensive or cause the woman any discomfort.

Micturition

Women should be asked if they are experiencing any problems associated with passing urine. It is abnormal for a woman to experience pain during micturition and this may be a sign of urinary tract infection. Women who report such pain should be asked for a midstream specimen of urine which should be sent to the laboratory for culture and sensitivity. Women often experience frequency of micturition during pregnancy because of the close proximity of the expanding uterus and bladder in early pregnancy, and the pressure of the fetal head in the third trimester. It is also common for women to experience some stress incontinence during pregnancy. This can be embarrassing and difficult for women to discuss. They should be reassured that they can help improve the tone of the pelvic floor by undertaking regular pelvic floor exercises (Hay-Smith et al 2001). Further research is required to evaluate the long-term efficacy of pelvic floor muscle training (Brostrom & Lose 2008).

Bowel function

Many pregnant women experience some alteration in their normal bowel habit when pregnant. The effect of progesterone on the smooth muscle of the bowel, further impeded by the gravid uterus, can lead to infrequent evacuation. Advice should include increasing water intake, eating additional fresh fruit and vegetables and a high fibre breakfast. Keeping active is also beneficial. If the woman is taking iron tablets it may be worth trying a different form. Aperients are only prescribed if these remedies fail, and should be of the bulk laxative variety (Jordan 2002).

Although less effective than laxatives that stimulate the bowel, they are less likely to cause abdominal discomfort or diarrhoea (Jewell & Young 1998). Haemorrhoids are exacerbated by constipation and may require treatment; the passage of hard stools will aggravate the haemorrhoids and the pain will make the woman reluctant to go to the toilet, thus worsening the constipation.

Dietary intake

The midwife should follow up women who were experiencing nausea and vomiting at booking. It is often assumed that once into the third trimester, this distressing symptom of pregnancy will have resolved. Unfortunately, this is not always the case and some women vomit throughout the pregnancy. Urinalysis for ketones is useful to ensure that the problem is not causing ketosis, which can make the woman feel even worse. Kind words and compassion go a long way to helping women cope and reassurance that the baby is not in danger is important.

Although weighing is not a routine aspect of antenatal care (NICE 2008), some women value being able to monitor their weight during pregnancy, but as a monitoring tool on its own, this has little clinical value.

Two-thirds of women suffer from heartburn in pregnancy (Enkin et al 2000), which can be painful, frequent and debilitating. Women will need advice about prevention, especially regarding keeping an upright posture, and alleviation of symptoms with prescribed antacids (remember there is no charge for prescriptions for pregnant women in the UK).

Skin integrity

Abdominal palpation to assess fetal growth is part of each antenatal examination (see Chapter 9). This provides the midwife with the opportunity to observe the integrity of the skin and identify any areas of concern. For example, the woman may have developed stretch marks (strai gravidarum) which can be red and intensely irritating. The woman can be reassured that they will fade over time, but unfortunately never completely disappear. The use of over-the-counter preparations can help minimize the appearance of these marks but there is no evidence that they can be prevented. The action of rubbing cream into affected areas will enhance the circulation and help keep the skin supple. Some women complain of intense itching during pregnancy. Where this is not associated with stretch marks or an obvious skin condition, this should be investigated to rule out obstetric cholestasis. Where itching is leading to intense scratching and sleepless nights, in the absence of a rash, liver function tests should be undertaken to rule out this condition (RCOG 2006).

Reflection on trigger scenario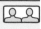

Look back on the trigger scenario.

Joanna is now 25 weeks pregnant. She has just returned from her antenatal check-up with the midwife. It was not the same midwife who had taken her booking history but she was friendly and took time to read through Jo's records. The midwife said that her blood pressure was up a bit, but when she retook it later it was fine. Jo had meant to ask her midwife what she should take for heartburn, but did not get the chance. She will call in at the chemist on her way to work.

The scenario highlights that women do not always see the same midwife throughout their pregnancy. This lack of continuity can be a source of dissatisfaction for some women, particularly when they have a complex history that they need to retell to numerous individuals. However, if the midwife is able to take time to get to know the woman, is respectful and listens attentively to the woman's story, the consultation can be a positive experience and mutually satisfying. Now that you are familiar with the physical examination of the mother during pregnancy you should have an insight into how the scenario relates to the evidence. The jigsaw model will now be used to explore the trigger scenario in more depth.

Effective communication

The midwife took time to read Jo's notes and get to know her, even though she had not met her before and may not meet her again. Annual leave and sickness can interfere with the best intentions to provide continuity of care for women. Questions that arise from the scenario might include: Where was the midwife who had undertaken the booking history? How can the midwife ensure that the details of the appointment are accurately conveyed to Jo's named midwife and to Jo? What forms of communication are used between professionals antenatally?

Woman-centred care

It is evident from the scenario that Jo liked the midwife and felt relaxed and respected. She had received some feedback about her blood pressure but this was rather vague. Questions that arise from the scenario might include: Did the midwife convey the actual blood pressure readings to Jo? Did Jo understand what the implications of raised blood pressure might have been? Did the midwife give any advice to Jo about what to do if she experienced any potential signs of pre-eclampsia? Did Jo leave the appointment feeling involved in her care? Jo had meant to ask about her heartburn but did not get the chance – how could this situation have been different?

Using best evidence

Raised blood pressure is a potential sign of pre-eclampsia, a condition with serious implications. It is essential that antenatal care is based on the best available evidence in order to detect and treat this life-threatening condition. Questions that arise from the scenario might include: What is the evidence to support the use of Korotkoff V as the diastolic blood pressure reading to record? Why did the midwife take Jo's blood pressure again? What is the most effective treatment for indigestion in pregnancy? What non-pharmacological measures can be taken to treat indigestion?

Professional and legal issues

The midwife was able to convey a demeanour that enabled Jo to feel confident in her hands. Questions that arise from the scenario might include: How did the midwife instil Jo with trust? What action does the midwife take to ensure that her practice remains up-to-date? Why is it essential to maintain legible, accurate records following each antenatal appointment? What action should the midwife take if she detects raised blood pressure in a woman during an antenatal clinic visit?

Team working

The midwife works as an autonomous practitioner within a team of healthcare professionals. She is the expert in the care of healthy pregnant women. Questions that arise from the scenario might include: Who can the community midwife call on if she detects an abnormality in a woman's pregnancy? How are relationships fostered and enhanced within the primary healthcare team? What processes are in place to ensure that general practitioners keep up-to-date with changes in protocols and guidelines? What is the role of the maternity care assistant in the care of pregnant women where you work?

Clinical dexterity

During the antenatal examination the midwife detected an elevation in Jo's blood pressure. Developing and maintaining this clinical skill is an essential part of the midwife's repertoire. Questions that arise from the scenario might include: What equipment is used in the community setting to measure blood pressure? Does the equipment in the hospital differ from that used in the hospital? Which arm should the midwife use to measure blood pressure? When was the sphygmomanometer last re-calibrated? How often should this be undertaken?

Models of care

Midwife-led care is the most appropriate model of care for women experiencing uncomplicated pregnancy. However, some women wish to have consultant-led care. Questions that arise from the scenario might include: Was Jo given a choice regarding the model of care she receives? Does she have a named midwife who has overall responsibility for her care? Does the midwife modify the schedule of care in the light of Jo's temporary raised blood pressure? Is there an audit of which professional is the lead carer for low-risk women?

Safe environment

The midwife detected an abnormality in Jo's blood pressure. She continued to care for Jo, undertaking the rest of her examination, before repeating the blood pressure measurement. She did not detect that Jo was suffering from heartburn. Questions that arise from the scenario might include: Is there sufficient flexibility in the maternity care system to spend extra time with women who need it? Was the clinic particularly busy that day? What must a midwife do if she feels that the environment of care is putting women at risk? Why did Jo not get the chance to ask about her heartburn? Are over-the-counter indigestion remedies safe for pregnant women?

Promotes health

Antenatal care provides an ideal opportunity to discuss healthy lifestyle practices that can influence the health of women and their families beyond this pregnancy. Questions that arise from the scenario might include: Did the midwife ask Jo if she had her blood pressure checked before she was pregnant? Did she inform Jo of the actual blood pressure reading so that Jo could take an active part in noting fluctuation in this measurement? If Jo had disclosed that she had troublesome heartburn, what advice might the midwife have offered?

Further scenarios

The following scenarios enable you to consider how specific situations influence the care the midwife provides. Use the jigsaw model to explore the issues raised in the scenario.

Scenario 1

Tracey is 30 weeks pregnant with her second baby. She has noticed that her feet and ankles are beginning to swell at the end of the day. This had not happened during her first pregnancy and she asks the midwife if there is anything she can take to get rid of the fluid. She comments that her auntie takes 'water tablets' for swollen legs.

Practice point

Further questions specific to Scenario 1 include:

1. Why do some women experience oedema during pregnancy?
2. Is oedema more prevalent in women expecting their second baby?
3. What advice can the midwife offer?
4. When will the oedema resolve?
5. Does the woman need referral to another health professional?

Scenario 2

Genevieve has had an uneventful pregnancy so far. She is now 35 weeks pregnant with her first baby. However, the last couple of nights' sleep have been disturbed with particularly itchy hands and feet, which she cannot stop scratching. Her mum recalls experiencing something similar when she was pregnant, but she does not remember anyone taking a great deal of notice at the time.

Practice point

Further questions specific to Scenario 2 include:

1. What are the possible causes of itching during pregnancy?
2. What are the risks of obstetric cholestasis for the mother and baby?
3. How is obstetric cholestasis diagnosed?

4. How is obstetric cholestasis usually monitored?

5. How is obstetric cholestasis usually managed?

Conclusion

Women may experience a range of emotions and physical changes throughout pregnancy. The student needs to adopt a thorough, yet not intrusive, approach to antenatal care. S/he will assess all aspects of maternal health during the antenatal check and take further agreed action where altered health is observed.

Resources

Action on pre eclampsia: http://www. apec.org.uk/.

Confidential Enquiry into Maternal and Child Health: http://www.cemach. org.uk/.

NHS Direct information about varicose veins: http://www.nhsdirect.nhs.uk/ articles/article.aspx?ArticleID=387#.

Obstetric Cholestasis Support Website: www.ocsupport.org.uk.

Pelvic floor exercises: http://www. continence-foundation.org.uk/ symptoms-and-treatments/pelvic-floor-exercises.php.

Women's Experiences of Maternity Care in the NHS in England: http://www. healthcarecommission.org.uk/_db/_ documents/Maternity_services_survey_ report.pdf.

References

Baston H, Hall J, Henley-Einion A: *Midwifery essentials: basics*, London, 2009, Elsevier.

Brostrom S, Lose G: Pelvic floor muscle training in the prevention and treament of urinary incontinence in women – what is the evidence?, *Acta Obstetrica et Gynecologica Scandinavica* 87(4): 384–402, 2008.

Enkin M, Keirse MJNC, Neilson J, et al: *A guide to effective care in pregnancy and childbirth*, ed 3, Oxford, 2000, Oxford University Press.

Hay-Smith E, Berghmans L, Hendriks H, et al: Pelvic floor muscle training for urinary incontinence in women, *Cochrane Database of Systematic Reviews* 1(CD001407), 2001.

Jewell D, Young G: Interventions for treating constipation in pregnancy, *Cochrane Database of Systematic Reviews* 3(CD001142), 1998.

Jordan S: *Pharmacology for midwives: the evidence base for safe practice*, Basingstoke, 2002, Palgrave.

Lewis G, editor: *The confidential enquiry into maternal and child health (CEMACH). Saving mothers' lives: reviewing maternal deaths to make motherhood safer – 2003–2005. The seventh report on confidential enquiries into maternal deaths in the United Kingdom*, London, 2007, CEMACH.

Melender HL, Lauri S: Security associated with pregnancy and childbirth – experiences of pregnant women, *Journal of Psychosomatic Obstetrics and Gynecology* 22(4): 229–239, 2001.

National Institute for Health and Clinical Excellence (NICE): *Antenatal care: routine care for the healthy pregnant woman: Clinical Guideline 62*, London, 2008, National Collaborating Centre for Women's and Children's Health.

RCOG: Obstetric cholestasis: Guideline 43, 2006. Online. Available http://www.rcog.org.uk/resources/Public/pdf/obstetric_cholestasis43.pdf April 27, 2008.

Redshaw M, Rowe R, Hockley C, et al: *Recorded delivery: a national survey of women's experience of maternity care*, Oxford, 2006, National Perinatal Epidemiology Unit.

Wheatley S: Psychosocial support in pregnancy. In Clement S, Page L, editors: *Psychological perspectives on pregnancy & childbirth*, Edinburgh, 1998, Churchill Livingstone.

Chapter 6

Monitoring women's emotional wellbeing in the antenatal period

Trigger scenario

Simone, a community based midwife, rings Joanna's doorbell. This is Joanna's first pregnancy and she is now 28 weeks pregnant. Joanna eventually opens the door. 'Hello,' Simone says. At which point Joanna bursts into tears. 'I am so scared,' she sobs.

Introduction

The onset of pregnancy will be a time of great joy for many women and their families. It will normally be a fulfilment of something that has been hoped for and wanted and a positive event in a woman's life. For other women a pregnancy may bring more negative emotions, especially in situations where it is unexpected or unplanned. However, most women will find that there will be a mixture of emotions over the course of the pregnancy, as it is a powerful, life-changing experience that affects the woman and those who are close to her. In an holistic approach to care it is important to think about the time of pregnancy in a complete way. How a woman will react in pregnancy will depend on many factors including her experiences before she became pregnant. Care will entail recognition of what is a natural emotional reaction to pregnancy in contrast to recognizing when reactions are pathological.

The World Health Organization web pages (WHO 2008a) state that:

Mental health is defined as a state of well-being in which every individual realizes his or her own potential, can cope with the normal stresses of life, can work productively and fruitfully, and is able to make a contribution to her or his community.

This means that part of a midwifery role will be to help women try to achieve this state. John Swinton (2001:35) has identified seven elements that define mental health:

- Absence of illness
- Appropriate social behaviour
- Freedom from worry and guilt
- Personal competence and control
- Self-acceptance and self-actualization
- Unification and organization of personality
- Open-mindedness and flexibility.

Activity

Think about yourself, and about how you feel in relation to the seven elements above. Decide which issues are relevant to you.

Consider the list above and relate it to the pregnant women in your care. Decide which issues are relevant to them at this time.

Emotional and mental wellbeing should be considered in an holistic way, recognizing the continuum between the body, mind and spirit (Davis-Floyd 2001). This means that what affects the physical part of a person will affect the other parts and vice versa.

The aim of this chapter is to consider emotional wellbeing in relation to pregnancy and to enable a midwife to provide women with support as they experience different emotions.

Background

Pregnancy is a time of change and adjustment. The changes that take place are physical, in that the fetus will be growing inside a woman and affecting her bodily processes. Amy Mullin (2002:38) writes that 'At no other time will an otherwise healthy adult undergo such widespread, rapid and undesired change in the shape and size of her body'. The changes will also be psychological, as she goes through adaptation into being a mother of this child (Rubin 1984, Raphael-Leff 1991, Mercer 1995). The profound nature of this change leads women to consider the experience as meaningful and spiritual (Carver & Ward 2007, Jesse et al 2007). It is important to recognize how the physical changes that take place in pregnancy can affect the emotional moods of women, and how psychological changes may also present with physical symptoms.

Hormonal influences

Activity

Remind yourself of the menstrual cycle and the changes in hormonal function in pregnancy. Think about how your mood changes throughout your menstrual cycle.

During pregnancy there are changes in circulating hormones in order to maintain the developing fetus. In the early weeks of pregnancy human chorionic gonadotrophin (HCG) is produced prior to the development of the placenta. During pregnancy the levels of oestrogens and progesterone rise with a subsequent effect on other normally produced hormones. Though a significant amount of research has been carried out on the effects of these hormones on mood, specifically in relation to the menstrual cycle and premenstrual syndrome, it has been shown that the levels of progesterone may have an effect in some women (Buckwalter et al 1999) but that the effect may be more indirect, in that they are combined with effects of stress, lack of social support and anxiety (Ross et al 2004). There is evidence to show that stress in pregnancy has some effect on the immune system and consequently may impact on the growth and development of the fetus (Coussons-Read et al 2003).

Physical changes

Physical changes take place in women during pregnancy, such as expanding waist lines, increase in hip and thigh and breast size. In addition she may also experience changes to her eyesight, skin pigments, blood pressure and breathing (Mullin 2002:39). A woman may experience symptoms in the course of the pregnancy of nausea or vomiting, fatigue, backache, heartburn, oedema or urinary or bowel changes that may have an influence on her feelings about herself. Certainly poor sleep quality in early pregnancy has been linked with

antenatal depression (Jomeen & Martin 2007). Physical illness in pregnancy, such as anaemia or hyperemesis gravidarum may lead to fatigue and less ability to adjust mentally (Cantwell & Cox 2003). An underactive thyroid gland may also lead to anxiety and depression (Timms 2007).

Activity

Ask someone who has a baby (or consider this if you have) how they felt about the changes that were taking place in their body.

Find out more about hyperemesis gravidarum, anaemia and underactive thyroid gland.

Body image

Changing identity during pregnancy also entails dealing with a changing body image (Mercer 1995:39). A woman's view of her body image prior to pregnancy will be related to her cultural views and the society in which she lives. For some women being pregnant and growing in size will make her feel better about herself (Price 1988:31). For others they may feel more negative about these changes (Stewart 2004:33, Lavender 2006). Current fashion promotes being thin as the ideal and such portrayal has been shown to be influential on pregnant women (Sumner et al 1993). Poor body image is linked to poor self-esteem and this may then be expressed through excessive dieting or purging of the body

(Lavender 2006). There is gathering evidence that poor nutritional status may have an influence on psychological wellbeing (Serci 2008). It has been shown that women may not be consuming enough of the appropriate nutrients in pregnancy (Thomas et al 2006). Exploration of a woman's diet in pregnancy should be made, especially if she has a low mood status.

Sexuality

The physical changes of the woman are also linked to her views of her sexual self. Jane Price (1988:31) writes: 'Pregnancy is a clear label both that the person is a woman and that she is sexually active.'

Her changing physical shape means that she is recognized by others as a sexual being (Mullin 2002:39). Pregnancy leads to changes of status in society with recognition that where she has previously been a daughter she is becoming a mother. This may be a complex state, particularly for some women who may feel uncomfortable about displaying their sexual selves and may choose to hide being pregnant for as long as possible. For others, being pregnant may heighten their sexual feelings (Raphael-Leff 1991:383).

Mary Stewart (2004:33) writes: 'women's bodies are likely to be touched more during and immediately after pregnancy than at any other time.'

A woman's concepts of her body and acceptance of being touched by 'strangers' will be linked to her emotional wellbeing in pregnancy.

Activity

Think about how you feel about being touched by strangers. Having reflected on this, think about how you could make your practice better to enable the women you look after to feel better about this.

More intensive aversion to being touched may be felt by women who are currently, or have been, in an abusive relationship. It could have a detrimental affect on women's mental health, and they will need specialist support, alongside careful midwifery care (Hobbins 2004, Baird 2007, Tiwari et al 2008).

Psychological changes

Significant changes take place psychologically in women and their partners over the course of pregnancy. Complex processes take place in relationships between partners and their wider family, as they adjust to the impending addition of a new family member (Raphael-Leff 1991, Mullin 2002:40). A woman's expectations and previous experiences of pregnancy will have a significant effect on how she copes and adapts to the changes that take place. These may be influenced by many factors, including how she has been brought up, the society and culture in which she resides and the social support she receives.

The process of adaptation often begins before pregnancy when couples make the decision to have a child. The reasons for this will be individual to the people involved, and sometimes will be subconscious (Bergum 1989, Raphael-Leff 1991). For women who were not expecting pregnancy the process of adaptation may take longer as they have to come to terms with the news (Marck 1994). Women who are experiencing a complicated pregnancy or have had a previous pregnancy loss may take a longer time to build a relationship with their unborn child, until the risk or threat to the pregnancy has passed, or they have passed the anniversary of the loss (Lever Hense 1994, McGeary 1994).

Current maternity provision in the UK includes opportunity for 'choice'. Women and their partners may have to make choices relating to place of birth, choice of caregiver and antenatal screening methods. Suggestion has been made that the introduction of screening may psychologically cause greater anxiety (Marteau 1989). Lorraine Sherr (1995) sums up as follows in relation to antenatal screening:

- May cause anxiety
- Delay in feedback may cause 'adverse emotional consequences'
- Poor communication skills may raise anxiety
- Anxiety may remain even after the outcomes have been negative or positive
- Medical practitioners are poor at identifying the nature of anxiety in women
- The widespread programmes make it difficult to respond to individual need and concern.

Activity

Think about your current experience of giving information about antenatal screening tests. In the light of the above information, work out whether there are ways this could be improved.

A recent study of the psychological effect of choice of place of birth has not shown that a particular type of care is of psychological benefit (Jomeen & Martin 2008).

Mercer's (1995:52) review of research relating to maternal identity has identified how women use fantasy and dreams during the process of change. It is suggested this is related to women mentally 'rehearsing' their future role as mother. Women may also experience grief and loss as they may lose some part of their identity through changing roles (Mercer 1995:59).

We can relate the change from non-mother to mother as a form of loss where women may have to reinterpret the ways in which they view themselves in accordance with their new role as a mother and caregiver, and revaluate their former self, as well as adjust to their new identity which is now on view to the wider society.

(Atkinson 2006)

This may be in relation to loss of status in leaving employment. It is common that women will express feelings of ambivalence, of 'not being ready' to have a baby during pregnancy, even if they have made a choice to become pregnant (Bergum 1989, Raphal Leff 1991:240).

Many women will experience anxiety at some point over pregnancy, however Lorraine Sherr (1995:137) suggests that anxiety may be a 'protective positive emotion' as a result of stressors. Problems may only arise should the anxiety be out of proportion to the stressors. Fears and anxieties relating to the wellbeing of the growing fetus are common. In Melender's (2002) survey of 329 pregnant women in Finland 78% of the respondents admitted to having some fear in relation to childbirth. The fears created different levels of stress and anxiety, which were more marked in those women experiencing their first pregnancy. The authors conclude by recommending that midwives should discuss a woman's fears in greater depth. A pathological condition of intense fear of childbirth has been defined and labelled tokophobia (Hofberg & Ward 2004) though Denis Walsh (2002) has challenged whether this is actually a 'normal' reaction to a traumatic event.

Hofberg and Ward (2003) state there are different types of tokophobia:

- Primary – when women have not had a baby before
- Secondary – where women have had previous traumatic deliveries
- Secondary to depressive illness in pregnancy.

Activity

Think about the three types of tokophobia mentioned. For each situation, decide how you as a midwife would support women.

Spirituality

Within an holistic philosophy of care, it is essential to consider the relevance of spirituality to the woman (Hall 2001). Pregnancy and childbirth is considered to be a powerful and meaningful event, which is a rite of passage into motherhood (Balin 1988, Wallas La Chance 1991, Ayers-Gould 2000). Spiritual and religious beliefs may become more significant during pregnancy, with these providing a source of coping with stressful situations (Carver & Ward 2007, Jesse et al 2007, Price et al 2007). The Royal College of Psychiatrists recognizes the significance of thinking about the spiritual dimension in relation to mental wellbeing (Royal College of Psychiatrists 2007). Spiritual care could lead to:

- Improved self-control, self-esteem and confidence
- Faster and easier recovery, achieved through both promoting the healthy grieving of loss and maximizing personal potential
- Improved relationships – with self, others and with God/creation/nature
- A new sense of meaning, resulting in reawakening of hope and peace of mind, enabling people to accept and live with problems not yet resolved.

This signifies that aiming to provide a spiritual focus to care may help women with emotional needs during pregnancy. The midwife may establish women's spiritual need by asking appropriate questions in the antenatal period (Hall, in press) and staying alert to signs of distress.

Antenatal depression

It has been suggested that pregnancy improves the condition of some women with psychiatric disorders. However, until recently, understanding of mental illness has been more focused on the postnatal period of childbirth than before birth. It has been identified that from 7.4–10.7% of women may have a type of antenatal depression in the first trimester of pregnancy with a potential 12.8% in the second trimester (Dennis et al 2007); whether this is as a result of pregnancy or has been present before pregnancy and gone undiagnosed is difficult to establish. Further, certain pre-existing psychiatric disorders may become worse in pregnancy (Hadwin 2007, Weeks 2007).

In Raymonds' (2007) study of some women's experience of antenatal depression it was identified that some found it hard to reveal their feelings and that it was common to feel 'emotional isolation'. The authors concluded this could have been helped through provision of continuity of carer. They further established that the partner may also have a need for support. The women identified helpful support mechanisms: massage, social groups, practical skill development and exercise plus access to web-based support groups.

In a Swedish study, Rubertsson et al (2005) showed that for those women who had signs of depression in the antenatal and postnatal period factors associated with this were:

- A difficult social situation, such as being unemployed, not having

Swedish as a first language and an unplanned or unwanted pregnancy
- Lack of social support, mostly from a partner but also from others
- Having experienced two or more stressful life events in the year prior to pregnancy
- Physical health issues during pregnancy and afterwards.

Rodriguez et al (2001) demonstrated that there may be a link between pregnancy symptoms experienced and psychological stress. The authors recommend that practitioners help to reduce stress in pregnancy. Difficult social situations that need to be considered include domestic violence, which may have a significant effect on the emotional wellbeing of the pregnant woman (Baird 2007).

Activity

With the knowledge of the above, think about how maternity services could be adapted to improve care of women. Decide what sort of information the midwife should find out.

National guidance

Mental health issues have been high on the government agenda for some time in the UK. The National Service Framework for Mental Health (Department of Health 1999) was one of the first to be produced and lays out the plans for mental health services in the UK. It includes the following standards:

Standard one

Health and social services should:

- Promote mental health for all, working with individuals and communities
- Combat discrimination against individuals and groups with mental health problems, and promote their social inclusion.

Standard two

Any service user who contacts their primary healthcare team with a common mental health problem should:

- Have their mental health needs identified and assessed
- Be offered effective treatments, including referral to specialist services for further assessment, treatment and care if they require it.

Standard three

Any individual with a common mental health problem should:

- Be able to make contact round the clock with the local services necessary to meet their needs and receive adequate care
- Be able to use NHS Direct, as it develops, for first-level advice and referral on to specialist helplines or to local services.

These standards apply to maternity services with the requirement for midwives to have a health promotion focus that considers how mental health may be promoted effectively in pregnant women (Hall 2007). Further, midwives should be able to recognize the needs of women with mental health challenges and be able to refer them to relevant services. The NICE (2008) Antenatal Guidelines gives guidance on antenatal questioning to establish those women who may have existing mental health conditions in pregnancy. Advice is also given about referral systems. NICE has also produced specific guidelines for women with existing mental health conditions (NICE 2007).

Activity

Access these guidelines from the NICE web pages and consider the relevance of the information to emotional health:
http://www.nice.org.uk/guidance/index.jsp?action=byType&type=2&status=3.

Professional regulation

The role of the midwife with regard to emotional health is clearly stated in a European Union Directive as one of the roles of midwives (NMC 2004:36):

To recognise the warning signs of abnormality in the mother or infant which necessitate referral to a doctor and to assist the latter where appropriate; to take the necessary emergency measures in the doctor's absence.

and student midwives are expected to learn to: 'refer women who would benefit from the skills and knowledge of other individuals.' (NMC 2009)

In this document it also states that midwives should: 'support the creation and maintenance of environments that promote the health, safety and wellbeing of women, babies and others.'

This indicates that thought should be given to the environments of maternity services and whether these have an impact on the mental wellbeing of women. Improving physical working environments through use of better design and use of art may have a positive effect on both staff and service users (Waller & Finn 2004). Giving better consideration to the environment of the maternity services is to be recommended (Newburn 2006). Considering where antenatal care takes place to ensure women feel safe to disclose sensitive information has been highlighted by NICE (2008:13).

In the NMC Code of conduct there is a clear instruction relating to women with mental illness:

You must be aware of legislation regarding mental capacity, ensuring that people who lack capacity remain at the centre of decision making and are fully safeguarded.

(NMC 2008:08)

The rules of practice indicate the responsibility of midwives to recognize when the issues of pregnancy deviate from 'normal' and to refer to appropriate specialists (NMC 2004:16).

Midwives role

In order to establish the needs of women, midwives should assess them appropriately. Asking the 'right'

questions and continual assessment through developing a relationship thoughout pregnancy is the ideal situation. Continuity of care may enable midwives to recognize emotional changes more quickly (Hall 2007:41).

Rubertsson et al's (2005) study suggests that a comprehensive 'psychosocial' history should be taken in early pregnancy that includes addressing:

- Previous mental health problems
- A woman's social support
- Stressful life events
- Employment status.

The WHO (2008b) also advises that questions should be asked in pregnancy and afterwards such as:

- Depression: 'How much of the time during the last month have you felt downhearted and blue?'
- Anxiety: 'How much of the time during the last month have you been a very nervous person?'
- Psychosis: 'Have you been receiving any special messages from people or from the way things are arranged around you?'

The NICE (2007) guidelines related to women with existing mental health conditions identify that at the first antenatal visit questions should be asked about:

- Past or present severe mental illness including schizophrenia, bipolar disorder, psychosis in the postnatal period and severe depression

- Previous treatment by a psychiatrist/ specialist mental health team including
  - inpatient care
  - a family history of perinatal mental illness.

And also, specifically in relation to depression:

- During the past month, have you often been bothered by feeling down, depressed or hopeless?
- During the past month, have you often been bothered by having little interest or pleasure in doing things?

A third question should be considered if the woman answers 'yes' to either of the initial questions.

- Is this something you feel you need or want help with?

The answers to these questions should help midwives establish if the women are having a 'normal' reaction to pregnancy or if there is some underlying mental health condition requiring referral. Definite identification of emotional or mental health disorders can be difficult to establish, therefore early referral may be the most appropriate option. Sandra Elliott et al (2007) identified that increased training of midwives in recognition of mental health issues enabled a much higher detection rate but that this also led to a greater pressure on referral services.

The best treatment for antenatal depression is not clear. A Cochrane review of psychosocial and psychological interventions (Dennis et al 2007)

only identified one study suitable and therefore concluded that evidence is insufficient to provide a recommendation. Discussions over medication for antenatal depression show that continuing treatment in pregnancy may be the most appropriate option (NICE 2007) balanced against the potential effect on the unborn baby.

Other mental conditions

NICE (2008) states that women with psychiatric conditions and addictive tendencies require more specialist care. These conditions include issues such as eating disorders, drug or alcohol addiction, bipolar disorder and obsessive disorder. The NICE (2007) Antenatal Mental Health Guidelines specifically cover care of such women. The midwife must acknowledge the limitations of her expertise and involve the wider multi-professional team in their care.

Reflection on trigger scenario

Look back to the scenario at the start of the chapter.

Simone, a community-based midwife, rings Joanna's doorbell. This is Joanna's first pregnancy and she is now 28 weeks pregnant. Joanna eventually opens the door. 'Hello,' Simone says. At which point Joanna bursts into tears. 'I am so scared,' she sobs.

This scenario describes a specific encounter during pregnancy. With the knowledge you now have about emotional changes in pregnancy you should be able to consider Joanna's situation and how a midwife may be able to help her. The jigsaw model will now be used to explore the situation in more depth.

Woman-centred care

Ensuring sensitive, individualized care for women means that midwives may be able to recognize when women need more intensive input from the midwife herself or from other health professionals. In this scenario the following could be asked: Is this a 'routine' visit or has it been instigated due to previous concerns about Joanna's wellbeing? Has she previously been included in plans about her care and asked what her needs are? Are her partner and family involved in her care? How does Joanna's experience at the moment relate to her expectations of this pregnancy? How will Simone include Joanna in the next aspects of her care?

Using best evidence

In this scenario the midwife needs to use the best evidence available to make decisions about the next aspects of her care. Questions that need to be addressed to ensure that the woman's care is evidence based include: What questions will Simone ask to establish what is happening to Joanna? What is the evidence concerning the causes of emotional distress in pregnancy? What evidence is there about appropriate forms of care or treatment? How will

Simone use National Guidelines to enable the most appropriate care for Joanna?

Professional and legal

Midwives should always practise within the framework of their profession and the law. In this scenario questions that need to be addressed to ensure that the woman's care fulfils statutory obligations include: Has Simone received enough appropriate training in relation to mental health issues? How do the rules of practice and NMC Code (2008) help her in Joanna's care? Are there any national or international guidelines relating to Joanna's care?

Team working

Though community based midwives often work alone they are also based within a primary health environment that involves other health professionals. Questions that need to be addressed in this scenario are: Are Joanna's needs significant to warrant inviting involvement of other professionals? If so, who will this be? Where will Simone record information for other health professionals? How will Simone make contact with other health professionals if required?

Effective communication

In caring for women during the antenatal period it is important to use appropriate communication skills, especially in relation to mental wellbeing. A midwife should especially listen to what a woman says and carefully observe her body language.

Questions that may be considered in this scenario are: Has Simone already developed a relationship with Joanna? Does she observe Joanna to be behaving differently? What questions should Simone ask about Joanna's feelings? What clues could be obtained from what and how Joanna replies? How should Simone record the discussion?

Clinical dexterity

In relation to emotional issues clinical skills may not usually be required, however if the midwife needs to carry out any tests following on from the discussion she should use sensitivity and gentleness. Questions that could arise are: Does Simone need to make any clinical assessments in relation to Joanna's care? Is this the appropriate time to carry out these assessments?

Models of care

In relation to antenatal care there are currently a number of models that midwives follow in the UK. How care is organized may have a positive or negative effect on the emotional wellbeing of some women. In this situation, questions that could be raised are: Does Simone work in a team of colleagues who aim to provide continuity through the whole pregnancy continuum? Would continuity be beneficial in this situation? Is home based care more beneficial in this situation? If so, why would this be? Are there other professional groups involved in the provision of the care Simone is giving?

Safe environment

All midwifery care should be carried out in a safe environment, for the woman, her family members and also for the midwife. Unpredictability of mental health issues means that midwives should be vigilant to ensure safety is maintained.

Questions that could be asked about this scenario are: Is Joanna in a safe environment in her home or are there reasons to believe she may be putting herself or her family at risk? Is Simone safe in visiting Joanna at home as a lone professional?

Promotes health

Antenatal care provides many opportunities for midwives to promote the emotional health of a woman, her family and the community in which they work. In this scenario questions that could be asked to ensure that the woman's care promotes health include: Does the environment where Joanna is living promote her mental wellbeing? Are there issues in the home that are damaging her health? Are there ways Simone could promote Joanna's emotional health at this time?

Further scenarios

The following scenarios enable you to consider how specific situations influence the care the midwife provides. Use the jigsaw model to explore the issues raised in each situation.

Scenario 1

Comfort has arrived at the antenatal clinic. She is 20 weeks pregnant and has just been transferred into the area as a refugee from a war-torn African country. She has arrived with her sister and two other children. Many of her family, including her partner and parents, are still in Africa. She speaks some English but does not always understand.

Practice point

Women who arrive as refugees may have considerable emotional needs. Not only are they living in strange, and often poor environments, many carry emotional scars of the experiences they have had in their homeland or of the journey they have had in getting to this country. Loss of family members or long-term separation may add to their burdens. Being able to access services may also be a challenge, as they may find it hard to understand our maternity system. Language difficulties may complicate understanding of needs on both sides and midwives need to be cautious in interpreting the emotional status of the woman before them.

Questions that could be asked in the care of Comfort are:

1. What feelings may Comfort be experiencing?
2. What effect could these have on the pregnancy?
3. What questions may the midwife ask her about her feelings?
4. Who should the midwife ask to provide translation if required?

5. What would be the most appropriate model of care?
6. How will the midwife ensure Comfort receives the best care to meet her needs?

Scenario 2

Carmel, a community midwife, receives a telephone call from the antenatal clinic to say that Anna, a woman on her caseload, has received a diagnosis of a fetal abnormality on an ultrasound. Anna intends to continue the pregnancy. Carmel promises to visit her at home.

Practice point

In a straightforward pregnancy the use of antenatal screening may cause a degree of anxiety. This will be heightened should there be a positive result. Choosing to continue with a pregnancy will be a difficult decision in an environment where there are expectations that women will choose to end it. Women and their family will need continual support in coming to terms with their fears, anxieties and grief of loss of expectations, as well as to build up a relationship with the unborn baby.

Questions sthat could be asked in the care of Anna are:

1. What communication skills will Carmel use when she is with Anna?
2. What sorts of questions will she ask?
3. What feelings may Anna be experiencing?
4. How will Carmel help Anna in her choice?
5. How may the partner and family be supported in this situation?

6. What model of care will be best during the rest of the pregnancy?

7. Which other professionals may be included in Anna's care?

Conclusion

Pregnancy brings changes to all aspects of a woman's life and in particular there are significant emotional and psychological adaptations that will take place. The midwife has an important role in recognizing the needs of women and helping meet those needs in an holistic way. She should also recognize when the psychological reactions are pathological and requiring referral to other professionals for further assessment and support.

Useful resources

Antenatal depression: Developing an effective and co-ordinated service: http://www.depression-in-pregnancy.org.uk/Antinatal%20depression%20book%20conversion.pdf.

MIND (National Association for Mental Health): http://www.mind.org.uk/.

National Collaborating Centre for Mental Health: *Antenatal and postnatal mental health: The NICE guideline on clinical management and service guidance.* London, 2007, NICE. Online. Available: http://www.nice.org.uk/guidance/index.jsp?action=download&o=30431.

National self harm network: http://www.nshn.co.uk/.

National Institute for Health and Clinical Excellence (NICE): Antenatal care: routine care for the healthy pregnant woman, London, 2008, NICE. Online. Available http://www.nice.org.uk/guidance/index.jsp?action=byID&o=11947.

Price SA, editor: *Mental health in pregnancy and childbirth*, Edinburgh, 2007, Churchill Livingstone.

Royal College of Psychiatrists: http://www.rcpsych.ac.uk/.

Self harm support web site: http://www.selfharm.net/.

References

Atkinson B: Gaining motherhood, losing identity, *MIDIRS Midwifery Digest* 16(2):170–174, 2006.

Ayers-Gould JN: Spirituality in birth: creating sacred space within the medical model, *International Journal of Childbirth Education* 15:14–17, 2000.

Baird K: Domestic abuse, violence and mental health. In Price SA, editor: *Mental health in pregnancy and childbirth*, Edinburgh, 2007, Churchill Livingstone.

Balin J: The sacred dimensions of pregnancy and birth, *Qualitative Sociology* 11:275–301, 1988.

Bergum V: *Woman to mother: a transformation*, Massachusetts, 1989, Bergin & Garvey.

Buckwalter JG, Stanczyk FZ, McCleary CA, et al: Pregnancy, the postpartum, and steroid hormones: effects on cognition and mood, *Psychoneuroendocrinology* 24:69–84, 1999.

Cantwell R, Cox JL: Psychiatric disorders in pregnancy and the puerperium, *Current Obstetrics and Gynaecology* 13:7–13, 2003.

Carver N, Ward B: Spirituality in pregnancy: a diversity of experiences and needs, *British Journal of Midwifery* 15(5):294–296, 2007.

Coussons-Read M, Okun M, Simms S: The psychneuroimmunology of pregnancy, *Journal of Reproductive and Infant Psychology* 21(2):103–112, 2003.

Davis-Floyd R: The technocratic, humanistic, and holistic paradigms of childbirth, *International Journal of Gynecology & Obstetrics* 75:S5–S23, 2001.

Dennis C-L, Ross LE, Grigoriadis S: Psychosocial and psychological inter-ventions for treating antenatal depression, *Cochrane Database of Systematic Reviews* 3(CD006309), 2007.

Department of Health: *National service framework for mental health: modern standards and service models*, London, 1999, Department of Health.

Elliott S, Ross-Davie M, Sarkar A, et al: Detection and initial assessment of mental disorder: the midwife's role, *British Journal of Midwifery* 15(12):759–764, 2007.

Hadwin P: Common mental health disorders. In Price SA, editor: *Mental Health in Pregnancy and Childbirth*, Edinburgh, 2007, Churchill Livingstone.

Hall J: *Midwifery, mind and spirit: emerging issues of care*, Oxford, 2001, Books for Midwives.

Hall J: Promoting mental well-being. In Price SA, editor: *Mental health in pregnancy and childbirth*, Edinburgh, 2007, Churchill Livingstone.

Hall J: Spirituality and labour care. In Walsh D, Downe S, editors: *Essential midwifery practice: intrapartum care*, Oxford, In press, Blackwell.

Hobbins D: Survivors of childhood sexual abuse: implications for perinatal nursing care, *Journal of Obstetric, Gynecological and Neonatal Nursing* 33:485–497, 2004.

Hofberg K, Ward MR: Fear of pregnancy and childbirth, *Postgraduate Medical Journal* 79:505–510, 2003.

Hofberg K, Ward MR: Fear of childbirth, tocophobia and mental health in mothers: the obstetric-psychiatric interface, *Clinical Obstetrics and Gynecology* 47(3):527–534, 2004.

Jesse DE, Schoneboom C, Blanchard A: The effect of faith or spirituality in pregnancy: a content analysis, *Journal of Holistic Nursing* 25(3):151–158, 2007.

Jomeen J, Martin CR: Assessment and relationship of sleep quality to depression in early pregnancy, *Journal of Reproductive and Infant Psychology* 25(1):87–99, 2007.

Jomeen J, Martin CR: The impact of choice of maternity care on psychological health outcomes for women during pregnancy and the postnatal period, *Journal of Evaluation in Clinical Practice* 14(3):391–398, 2008.

Lavender V: Body image: change, dissatisfaction and disturbance. In Price SA, editor: *Mental health in pregnancy and childbirth*, Edinburgh, 2006, Churchill Livingstone.

Lever Hense A: Livebirth following stillbirth. In Field PA, Marck PB, editors: *Uncertain motherhood: negotiating the risks of the childbearing years*, London, 1994, Sage Publications.

Marck PB: Unexpected pregnancy: the uncharted land of women's experience. In Field PA, Marck PB, editors: *Uncertain motherhood: negotiating the risks of the childbearing years*, London, 1994, Sage Publications.

Marteau T: Psychological cost of screening, *BMJ* 299(6698):527, 1989.

McGeary K: The influence of guarding on the developing mother-unborn child relationship. In Field PA, Marck PB, editors: *Uncertain motherhood: negotiating the risks of the childbearing years*, London, 1994, Sage Publications.

Melender H-L: Experiences of fears associated with pregnancy and childbirth: a study of 329 pregnant women, *Birth* 29:101–111, 2002.

Mercer RT: *Becoming a mother: research on maternal identity from Rubin to the present*, New York, 1995, Springer Publishing.

Mullin A: Pregnant bodies, pregnant minds, *Feminist Theory* 3(1):27–44, 2002.

National Collaborating Centre for Mental Health: *Antenatal and postnatal mental health: The NICE guideline on clinical management and service guidance*. London, 2007, NICE. Online. Available http://www.nice.org.uk/guidance/index.jsp?action=download&o=30431 March 2, 2008.

Newburn M: Curtains for the old delivery suite, *The Practising Midwife* 9(1):12–14, 2006.

National Institute for Health and Clinical Excellence (NICE): Antenatal care: routine care for the healthy pregnant woman. Online. Available http://www.nice.org.uk/guidance/index.jsp?action=byID&o=11947 April 4, 2008.

Nursing and Midwifery Council (NMC): *Midwives rules and standards*, London, 2004, NMC.

Nursing and Midwifery Council (NMC): *The code. Standards of conduct, performance and ethics for nurses and midwives*, London, 2008, NMC.

Nursing and Midwifery Council (NMC): *Standards for pre-registration midwifery education*, London, 2009, NMC.

Price J: *Motherhood: what it does to your mind*, London, 1988, Pandora.

Price S, Lake M, Breen G, et al: The spiritual experience of high-risk pregnancy, *Journal of Obstetric, Gynecologic and Neonatal Nursing* 36:63–70, 2007.

Raphael-Leff J: *Psychological processes of childbearing*, Edinburgh, 1991, Chapman Hall.

Raymonds JE: 'Creating a safety net': women's experiences of antenatal depression and their identification of helpful community support and services during pregnancy, 2007. Online. Available http://www.sciencedirect.com/science?_ob=ArticleURL&_udi=B6WN9-4NCKK3S-1&_user=10&_rdoc=1&_fmt=&_orig=search&_sort=d&view=c&_acct=C000050221&_version=1&_urlVersion=0&_userid=10&md5=1f0585e374ef2253d47271e7e788538c December 1, 2008.

Rodriguez A, Bohlin G, Lindmark G: Symptoms across pregnancy in relation to psychosocial and biomedical factors, *Acta Obstetrica Et Gynecologica Scandinavica* 80(3):213–223, 2001.

Ross LE, Sellers EM, Gilbert Evans SE, et al: Mood changes during pregnancy and the postpartum period: development of a biopsychosocial model, *Acta Psychiatrica Scandinavica* 109(6):457–466, 2004.

Royal College of Psychiatrists: *Spirituality and mental health*. Online. Available http://www.rcpsych.ac.uk/mentalhealthinformation/therapies/spiritualityandmentalhealth.aspx March 3, 2008, London, 2007, Royal College of Psychiatrists.

Rubertsson C, Walderstrom U, Wickberg B, et al: Depressive mood in early pregnancy and postpartum: prevalence and women at risk in a national Swedish sample, *Journal of Reproductive and Infant Psychology* 23(2):155–166, 2005.

Rubin R: *Maternal identity and the maternal experience*, New York, 1984, Springer.

Serci I: Midwifery basics: diet matters (6). Perinatal mental health: relationships with diet and nutrition, *The Practising Midwife* 11(4):37–40, 2008.

Sherr L: *The psychology of pregnancy and childbirth*, Oxford, 1995, Blackwell Science.

Stewart M: Feminisms and the body. In Stewart M, editor: *Pregnancy, birth and maternity care: feminist perspectives*, Oxford, 2004, Elsevier.

Sumner A, Waller G, Killick S, et al: Body image distortion in pregnancy: a pilot study of the effects of media images, *Journal of Reproductive and Infant Psychology* 11:203–208, 1993.

Swinton J: *Spirituality in mental health care: rediscovering a forgotten dimension*, London, 2001, Jessica Kingsley Publishers.

Thomas B, Ghebremeskel K, Lowy C, et al: Nutrient intake of women with and without gestational diabetes with a specific focus on fatty acids, *Nutrition* 22:230–236, 2006.

Timms P: *Physical illness and mental health*. Online. Available http://www.rcpsych.ac.uk/mentalhealthinformation/mentalhealthproblems/physicalillness/copingwithphysicalillness.aspx March 25, 2008, London, 2007, Royal College of Psychiatrists.

Tiwari A, Chan KL, Fong D, et al: The impact of psychological abuse by an intimate partner on the mental health of pregnant women, *BJOG: An*

International Journal of Obstetrics and Gynaecology 115(3):377–384, 2008.

Wallas La Chance C: *The way of the mother: the lost journey of the feminine*, London, 1991, Vega.

Waller S, Finn H: *Enhancing the healing environment: a guide for NHS trusts*, London, 2004, King's Fund.

Walsh D: Fear of labour and birth, *British Journal of Midwifery* 10(2):78, 2002.

Weeks NP: Serious mental illness and the midwife. In Price SA, editor: *Mental health in pregnancy and childbirth*, Edinburgh, 2007, Churchill Livingstone.

World Health Organization: WHO urges more investments, services for mental health, 2008a. Online. Available http://www.who.int/mental_health/en/ March 20, 2008.

World Health Organization: Maternal mental health & child health and development, 2008b. Online. Available http://www.who.int/mental_health/prevention/suicide/MaternalMH/en March 20, 2008.

Chapter 7

Blood tests in pregnancy

Trigger scenario

Joanna is now 30 weeks pregnant. She has been feeling particularly tired and her mum suggested that she might be anaemic. Louis is rather insulted as he prides himself on buying the best fresh ingredients from the local market, they love cooking and eat plenty of fruit and vegetables. Joanna had a full blood count taken by the community midwife who came to the flat to do her booking history.

Introduction

Pregnancy is a time when women are faced with many choices and decisions. There is a plethora of information about why various tests are being made, but it does not always reach those women who need it most. An important aspect of the student midwife's progression from novice to competent practitioner is the development of an ability to present information to women in a meaningful manner, in a way that makes sense to them. As well as developing the necessary communications skills and self-awareness to approach women with confidence and competence, the student needs to feel that s/he has a firm underpinning knowledge of the facts. Being a student is challenging. Just as you thought you were getting to grips with a subject, a new dimension emerges. As you become familiar with one policy another is produced to take its place. Change is a constant factor in professional life, but an understanding of key principles provides a stable base from which new approaches can be explored.

This chapter considers the routine blood tests offered in pregnancy (Table 7.1). Although women may be advised to undergo such blood tests, they should not be pressured or coerced. It must also be noted that some maternity units offer different tests at different times, depending on local policy and the needs of the local community. Antenatal screening for fetal abnormality, including inherited disorders, will be considered separately in Chapter 8.

Midwives involved in taking blood from pregnant women need to consider the following:

- Occasionally some women do not want to have what are considered by professionals to be 'routine' tests. They have a right to decline. Although you have a responsibility to inform them of the consequences of their decision and to document that you have done so, take a non-judgmental approach. As a student, you must always refer any controversy or uncertainty to a registered professional.

- Just because there is a lot of information to absorb during pregnancy, does not mean that women do not want to receive it.

- Some women have needle phobia and need to be treated with sensitivity.

- Some women faint when they have blood taken – always ask a woman if this is the case!

- See *Midwifery Essentials: Basics*, Chapter 9: Venepuncture, for the procedure for taking blood.

The booking history was explored in Chapter 3. It was seen that a detailed account of the woman's current health, previous medical, social and obstetric history is taken in order to identify potential factors that might impact on the woman's or her baby's wellbeing. Taking maternal blood is another procedure that enables further risk factors to be identified or potential pathology avoided.

The sooner that these important blood tests are taken, the sooner results can be acted upon. NICE guidance (NICE 2008) recommends that the booking appointment takes place by week 10 of the pregnancy. However, when blood is taken from women depends on the model of care in operation and on the local services available. Some community midwives who undertake the booking history in the community also take the booking bloods at the same time. It is important that there is a system to ensure safe transportation of these blood samples to the local laboratory, which is usually situated in the hospital Trust. The midwife will often make her booking appointments in the morning so that the samples can meet the pick-up service that serves the general practitioner's surgery or health centre that she links with. Where such services do not exist, women attend the hospital for booking bloods, usually at the same time as the first scan. In some areas, the practice nurse takes blood, after appropriate counselling by the midwife, and there is a local arrangement for samples to be taken at a time that coincides with other clinics.

Whoever takes the blood, or requests that it is taken by someone else, should ensure that the result is followed up and documented in the appropriate place. The National Maternity Record has a dedicated page for the documentation of blood test results.

Activity

Make sure you know what a phlebotomist is.

Find out if there is a phlebotomy service at the Trust where you work.

Think about when women have their booking bloods taken in your locality, and who normally takes them.

Blood tests in pregnancy

For a summary of the blood tests routinely offered in pregnancy, see Table 7.1.

Full blood count

The full blood count is taken to identify maternal anaemia with the aim of

Table 7.1 Routine blood tests offered during pregnancy

Blood test	Who	When
Full blood count (FBC)	All	Booking and third trimester
Hepatitis B virus (HBV)	All	Booking
Blood group and rhesus factor	All	Booking
Rhesus antibody screening	Rhesus negative women	28 weeks
Red cell alloantibodies	All	Booking and 28 weeks
Rubella antibodies	All	Preconceptually or booking
Syphilis (VDRL)	All	Booking
Human immunodeficiency virus (HIV)	All	Booking
Maternal serum screening for Down's syndrome (see Chapter 8)	All	Combined test at 11 + 0 days–13 weeks + 6 days. Triple/Quad test 15–20 weeks
Sickle cell anaemia	Women (or those with partners or relatives) from Africa, Mediterranean, Far/Middle East, Asia and Caribbean	Booking
Thalassaemia (see Chapter 8)		Booking

Table 7.2 The full blood count in relation to pregnancy

Test	What	Normal (women)	Pregnancy
Haemoglobin (Hb)	Amount of haemoglobin in the blood measured in grams per decilitre: g/dL or g/100ml	12.5–15.5	Falls 2g until about 30 weeks (steepest drop by 20 weeks) then rises slightly to term
Red cell count (RCC)	Number of red cells per litre of blood: $\times 10^{12}$ per litre	4.2–4.5	Falls by about 1 until 30–34 weeks
Haematotcrit (Hct) of packed cell volume (PCV)	Percentage of blood cells to total blood volume	35–45	Falls by about 6% until 30 weeks then rises slightly to term
Mean corpuscular (cell) volume (MCV)	An estimated volume of indivdual red blood cells (fL)	80–100	Increase in macrocytic anaemia Decrease in microcytic anaemia
Mean cell haemoglobin (MCH)	Haemoglobin content within erythrocyte of average size (pg)	27–32	Increase in macrocytic anaemia Decrease in microcytic anaemia
Red cell mass	Total volume of red blood cells in the circulation	1400	Up to 1650 by term
White cell count (WCC)	Total number of white blood cells in the circulation	4–11	May be raised up to 15
Platelets	Number of platelets per litre of blood ($\times 10^3$) per mm^3	150–400	Slight decrease

Sources include: Luckman & Sorensen (1980); Chamberlain & Morgan (2002); Shuttleworth (2002); Stables & Rankin (2005)

treating the condition, if necessary. However, it also provides a useful picture of the woman's current health status in many more respects (see Table 7.2). For example, a fall in platelets may be seen in women who develop pre-eclampsia, and a raised white cell count may be indicative of underlying infection. In some trusts, serum ferritin levels are also measured as they reflect the woman's iron reserves and fall before haemoglobin levels.

It is normal for a woman's haemoglobin to fall in pregnancy and this reflects an expansion in plasma volume which exceeds the increase in red cell mass. A failure of the haemoglobin concentration to fall has been linked with an increase in the incidence of preterm birth and low birthweight (Steer et al 1995). Stephansson et al (2000), in a matched case-control study, found an association between high first haemoglobin and increased risk of stillbirth. The National Institute for Health and Clinical Excellence (NICE 2008) recommend that a haemoglobin level of less than 11 g per decilitre (g/100 ml) at booking and below 10.5 g/100 ml at 28 weeks should be investigated and iron supplementation considered. Barrett et al (1994) argue that during normal pregnancy, the woman increases her absorption of iron from her diet and this adaptation is sufficient to meet the requirements of pregnancy if her diet is adequate. There are many issues regarding correct diagnosis of iron deficiency anaemia (Coggins 2001). According to Enkin et al (2000:43):

an individual's haemoglobin concentration depends much more on the complex relation between red-cell mass and plasma volume than on deficiencies of iron or folate.

It is suggested that mean corpuscular volume (MCV) is a better indicator of iron deficiency (Stables & Rankin 2005): it falls during iron deficiency anaemia and is higher in folic acid deficiency anaemia (Bewley 2004). However, further research

is required to account for potential confounding by the macrocytic effect of folate deficiency (Steer et al 1995). Reveiz et al (2007), in a systematic review of the evidence regarding the treatment of iron deficiency anaemia in pregnancy, did not find any conclusive evidence as to when or how it should be treated.

Activity

Find out what is meant by 'haemolytic anaemia' and 'haemorrhagic anaemia'. Make sure you can identify the signs and symptoms of iron deficiency anaemia. Find out how much the plasma volume increases in pregnancy. Consider how anaemia is treated where you work.

Blood group and rhesus factor

The batch of blood samples taken at the booking appointment include blood group and rhesus factor. There are four blood groups and each may be either rhesus positive or negative, giving eight different types in total (see Table 7.3).

Table 7.3 Blood groups

Group	Rhesus +	Rhesus −
A	A +	A −
B	B +	B −
AB	AB +	AB −
O	O +	O −

It is important to know the woman's blood group in the event that she might require an emergency blood transfusion. However, when it is anticipated that a woman might need a blood transfusion, during a caesarean section or following a post-partum haemorrhage, for example, a blood sample will be taken so that her blood and donor blood can be 'cross-matched' in the laboratory, to ensure compatibility of the transfused blood with the woman's blood.

Identifying a woman's rhesus factor is important during pregnancy for the 15% of women who are rhesus negative. If blood from a rhesus negative person mixes with blood from a rhesus positive person, rhesus antibodies will be formed. If this happens again, the body is already armed to fight the invasion of a foreign factor, and haemolysis occurs. Consider that a rhesus negative woman is carrying a rhesus positive baby. If some of the baby's blood transfers across the placenta into her bloodstream, after approximately 72 hours she will develop rhesus antibodies. On this occasion there is little consequence; however, if the woman were to become pregnant again with a rhesus positive baby, antibodies would already be present and able to cross the placenta causing haemolysis of the fetal red blood cells (erythrocytes). The potential for harm depends on the degree of haemolysis. The developing baby may become anaemic through the development of this condition known as 'haemolytic disease of the newborn' (HDN). This is a potentially fatal condition: the fetus may develop heart failure 'hydrops fetalis' or if born alive, severe jaundice. Rhesus negative women should have their rhesus antibody status checked in early pregnancy and again at 28 weeks' gestation. For a summary of how the development of rhesus antibodies can be prevented, see Box 7.1.

Activity

Situations that increase the likelihood of blood from the fetus entering the maternal bloodstream are known as 'sensitizing events'. Identify five such events.

Box 7.1 Prevention of rhesus antibodies

Development of rhesus antibodies by the mother can be prevented if:

- the sensitizing event is known
- the significance of the event is realized
- the event is reported
- the practitioner acts on the knowledge
- Anti-D immunoglobulin is administered within 72 hours of the event
- prophylactic anti-D is administered during pregnancy.

Anti-D

If a sensitizing event is known, reported and confirmed within 72 hours an intramuscular injection of anti-D immunoglobulin can be given to the woman to prevent her from making antibodies in response to the feto-maternal transfusion (fmt). Such an event can be confirmed and quantified by the Kleihauer test or the more accurate flow cytometry (RCOG 2002).

The administration of anti-D following sensitizing events was introduced in 1969. Anti-D is administered to rhesus negative women who give birth to a rhesus positive baby to prevent iso-immunization causing haemolytic disease of the newborn in a subsequent pregnancy. This process has been very successful and now the most vulnerable time for iso-immunization is feto-maternal transfusion in pregnancy where there has been no obvious sensitizing event. In 2002, therefore, it was recommended that anti-D should be administered to RhD-negative women to prevent sensitization: routine anti-D prophylaxis (RAADP) (NICE 2002). This guidance stated that all non-sensitized rhesus negative pregnant women should receive anti-D at 28 weeks' and 34 weeks' gestation and was supported by the Royal College of Obstetricians and Gynaecologists (RCOG 2002) clinical green top guidance (No. 22). Whilst it is acknowledged that such administration of anti-D does reduce the incidence of iso-immunization (Crowther 2002) there is also the practice

issue that many women who have potentially sensitizing events are not being offered anti-D (McSweeney et al 1998). The Royal College of Midwives, in a communication in response to the publication of the guidance from NICE, also highlight the issue of informed choice for women and the need for women to be better informed about potentially sensitizing events (RCM 2002). The National Institute for Health and Clinical Excellence (NICE 2008) continues to recommend the administration of two doses of prophylactic anti-D for rhesus negative women.

It must be noted that there is a small but potential risk of anaphylaxis following administration and the complexity of administering it safely during pregnancy. Also, live vaccines should not be administered within 3 months of administration of anti-D as it will render them inactive (Jordan 2002). Anti-D can be given at the same time as the measles, mumps and rubella vaccine (MMR) using separate syringes and contralateral limbs, in the postnatal period (NHS Immunisation information

Activity

Find out how RAADP is being implemented where you work. If midwives routinely offer anti-D to non-sensitized rhesus negative women, find out where it is administered during pregnancy and by whom. Make sure you can recognize the signs of anaphylaxis.

2007). Women who are already sensitized should not receive anti-D.

Red cell antibodies

There is also the potential for women to make antibodies in response to exposure to any foreign blood, either following sensitization from paternal red cell antigens or through a previous blood transfusion (UK blood transfusion and tissue transplantation service 2007a). Antibody screening should therefore be performed on all samples used for antenatal and pre-transfusion testing (UK blood transfusion and tissue transplantation service 2007b). This applies to all women irrespective of their rhesus status and should be performed in early pregnancy and again at 28 weeks' gestation (NICE 2008). Such testing enables the presence of antibodies to be picked up and then the identification of the specific antibody where appropriate. This process is important because some antibodies are more clinically significant than others: anti-D, anti-C and Anti-Kell are all capable of causing severe haemolytic disease of the newborn (UK blood transfusion and tissue transplantation service 2007a). When a woman of blood group O with immunoglobulin anti-A and anti-B is pregnant with a baby of blood group A or B, there is the potential for HDN to develop: known as 'ABO incompatibility'. When a clinically significant red cell antibody is identified, the woman should be offered further investigation at a specialist centre (NICE 2008). Where one of these antibodies is identified it is useful to have access to test the blood of the baby's father, although in some cases this may be difficult to action.

Activity

Consider the blood tests in Table 7.1. Find out what forms and bottles are used for each test, and which laboratory each one is sent to.

Rubella antibodies

Antibodies to rubella (German measles) develop either as a result of natural exposure to the infection or through immunization. However, continued immunity is not guaranteed and rubella antibody status is checked preferably before, but usually early in each pregnancy.

Primary rubella infection is associated with the development of serious fetal abnormalities, including deafness, heart defects and encephalopathy. Hull & Johnston (1993) state that 85% of babies exposed to the infection in the first 8 weeks of pregnancy will have congenital abnormality. Women exposed to others with a rubella type rash, or indeed if they themselves develop such a rash, should seek medical advice, unless known to be rubella immune. Blood assays for rubella specific IgM/IgG in association with clinical information are required to assess the individual risk, although caution should be taken in interpreting results (Best et al 2002).

It is recommended that women are immunized following the birth if they were shown not to be rubella immune during pregnancy. It is recommended that women are not immunized during pregnancy nor that they become pregnant within 2 months after vaccination (Symonds & Symonds 2004) due to the concern that the live vaccine may be teratogenic. However, there have not been any reported cases of congenital rubella following inadvertent immunization to a pregnant women (Advisory Committee on Immunization Practices (ACIP) 2001).

Syphilis (VDRL)

Women have been routinely tested for syphilis at the booking appointment for many years and its incidence in Britain is now rare. However, there are examples of outbreaks, for example between 1997–2000, four outbreaks were recorded in the United Kingdom by the Public Health Laboratory Service (PHLS 2001). Untreated syphilis may result in prematurity, perinatal death, congenital lesions and deformities. However, it can be treated with penicillin and its detection and treatment can prevent the baby from being born with congenital syphilis.

Human immunodeficiency virus (HIV)

A joint press release from the Royal College of Midwives and the Department of Health in 1999 (Royal College of Midwives/Department of Health Joint Press Release 1999) urged midwives to give women an informed choice about taking up the opportunity for HIV testing in pregnancy. It arose because it was apparent that many women who gave birth while they were HIV infected did not know that they had the infection. They could not, therefore, seek measures that could reduce the risk of infecting their baby by avoiding breastfeeding and the use of antiretroviral treatment. Connor et al (1994) reported that without treatment the mother to child transmission occurs in 25.5% of births and this incidence was reduced to 8% with antiretroviral treatment with zidovudine. The RCOG (2004) report a 15–20% mother to child transmission in non-breastfeeding HIV positive women. It is reported by the National Study of HIV in pregnancy (NSHPC 2007) that 30 infants are infected annually within the UK. The national screening committee continues to recommend that all pregnant women should be offered HIV testing in early pregnancy (National Screening Committee 2007).

Offering HIV screening to all women has had considerable implications for maternity services and the midwives who deliver care. Midwives have developed and attended programmes of education to enable them to provide a sensitive and effective service, both for those who agree to be tested and those who decline. A positive result impacts not only on the woman and her unborn baby, but on her partner, family and friends. Women who test positive for HIV should be managed by a multi-professional team (RCOG 2004).

Hepatitis B virus (HBV)

Hepatitis literally means 'inflammation of the liver' and is caused by a viral infection. Some individuals never show signs of acute infection although it is usual for some degree of fever, loss of appetite and general malaise to precede jaundice. For others the acute infection is severe and potentially fatal. Following infection, symptoms may last for several weeks and relapse may also occur. Individuals may then become carriers of the virus. The principal mode of transmission is by exposure to blood or blood products, and a mother can pass it to her baby. If a woman's viral status is known, however, her baby can receive a course of immunization that can help prevent the development of carrier status. It was recommended (NHS Executive 1998, RCM 1999) that all pregnant women should be offered HBV screening, irrespective of their potential risk. The National Institute for Health and Clinical Excellence continues to recommend screening for HBV in all pregnancies. However, it does not support routine testing for hepatitis C as there is currently insufficient evidence regarding the effectiveness and cost benefits (NICE 2008).

Activity

Given that HBV transmission is via body fluids, think about who you would expect to be particularly vulnerable to this infection. Describe what jaundice is. Find out what is meant by 'icterus'.

Reflection on trigger scenario

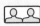

Look back on the trigger scenario

Joanna is now 30 weeks pregnant. She has been feeling particularly tired and her mum suggested that she might be anaemic. Louis is rather insulted as he prides himself on buying the best fresh ingredients from the local market, they love cooking and eat plenty of fruit and vegetables. Joanna had a full blood count taken by the community midwife who came to the flat to do her booking history.

Now that you are familiar with the schedule of blood tests in pregnancy, you should have insight into how the scenario relates to the evidence about detecting iron deficiency anaemia. The jigsaw model will now be used to explore the trigger scenario in more depth.

Effective communication

It is essential that midwives communicate effectively with women to ensure that they can provide informed consent for the blood tests on offer. A robust and clear system of communicating blood results is also key to effective care in pregnancy. Questions that arise from the scenario might include: Did the midwife inform Joanna how she would let her know if she was anaemic? Where did the hard copy of the results go to? Is there a computer system that would enable the midwife to quickly access Joanna's results if Joanna contacted her about them? Was the result recorded in Joanna's notes at a subsequent antenatal appointment?

Woman-centred care

All women need to feel that they understand the implications of the tests on offer if they are to participate fully in their care. They need to feel able to ask questions about how a particular test might be relevant to their individual situation. Questions that arise from the scenario might include: Were particular tests highlighted as being particularly relevant to Joanna? Did she feel that the tests were all routine and that she had no say in whether or not she wanted them? Did Joanna feel that her results would be conveyed to her, whether or not any action was required following the results?

Using best evidence

Routinely performing blood tests on pregnant women has significant resources implications, not only in terms of financial cost but also in terms of the midwife's time. It is important therefore that unnecessary tests are not performed and that those that are routine are based on best evidence. Questions that arise from the scenario might include: What processes are followed when the National Institute for Health and Clinical Excellence writes a new or reviews its previous guidance? How is that information made available to professionals? Who disseminates this information where you work? What do NICE guidelines say about testing for and treating anaemia in pregnancy?

Professional and legal issues

Taking blood from women during pregnancy has many professional and legal implications. It is essential that midwives keep up-to-date with current practice and new local and national guidance. The rationale behind the various tests that midwives take is not always made explicit. Questions that arise from the scenario might include: Do you feel able to counsel a woman who requires a full blood count during pregnancy? Do you always inform women about the implications of an abnormal result? What does the NMC say about keeping your skills and knowledge up-to-date? Where do you document the results of blood tests taken?

Team working

There are many professionals involved in the care of pregnant women. Midwives rely on the development and maintenance of effective working relationships with all those who input into their care. Questions that arise from the scenario might include: How many professionals are involved in taking blood, undertaking the analysis, reporting the result and taking any required action based on the findings? Who else is able to take blood where you work? Whose responsibility is it to find out the results of a blood test taken by you? Does the woman have any responsibility?

Clinical dexterity

Taking blood requires considerable clinical dexterity, not only to handle the equipment but also to find the most appropriate vein for venepuncture and disposing of the contaminated sharps.

Questions that arise from the scenario might include: How did you learn to take blood? Do you follow Trust guidance and always wear gloves when taking blood from women? Have you picked up any helpful tips by watching other professionals take blood? What are the challenges of taking blood in a woman's home?

Models of care

When blood is taken from a woman it is important that it makes its way to the laboratory without delay. Different models of care require specific systems to be in place to ensure that blood arrives safely in the laboratory. Questions that arise from the scenario might include: How does blood taken in the hospital get from the ward or clinic to the laboratory? What are the collection times or is there an automated chute system? If blood is taken in the community, how does it get from the woman's home to the laboratory? Is this system effective?

Safe environment

Taking blood from a woman poses potential risks to anyone coming into that environment. For the woman the risks include: infection, haematoma and incorrect identification. Questions that arise from the scenario might include: Did the blood sample arrive safely in the laboratory for testing? How do you follow up the results of blood that you have taken or requested? Do you have any knowledge of the impact on the laboratory staff of receiving an

inappropriately labelled blood sample? What is the procedure if this happens?

Promotes health

Every contact that a midwife has with a pregnant woman is an opportunity to improve her general health and wellbeing. In addition to the public health benefits of counselling her regarding healthy eating to avoid or treat anaemia, treating her with kindness and respect will have a long-lasting impact on her emotional wellbeing. Questions that arise from the scenario might include: Did the midwife ask Joanna about her diet when she was taking blood to screen for anaemia. Did the midwife inform Joanna of sources of iron rich food and the added benefit of consuming them in conjunction with vitamin C to enhance absorption?

Further scenarios

The following scenarios enable you to consider how specific situations influence the care the midwife provides. Use the jigsaw model to explore the issues raised in each scenario.

Scenario 1

Tessa is 34 weeks pregnant. She has just been to the local primary school to pick up her daughter from nursery. She overhears a group of women saying that there are two children in the school with suspected German measles. She remembers reading in one of her pregnancy books that there is a possible danger for unborn babies if their mother comes into contact with the virus.

Practice point

Further questions specific to Scenario 1 include:

1. When in pregnancy are women tested for the rubella immunity status?
2. How is this result conveyed to women?
3. What action would you take if Tessa contacted you as her midwife for advice?
4. When is infection with rubella particularly hazardous for the unborn baby?
5. What public health measures are taken to reduce the incidence of rubella infection in the community?

Scenario 2

Catherine wants a home birth. She had an uneventful first labour and birth and really wants to avoid going into hospital if at all possible. Her community midwife has informed her that local policy requires her to have a haemoglobin above 10.5 g/100 ml at the onset of labour. She is currently 30 weeks' pregnant and her last haemoglobin was only 9.8 g/100 ml.

Practice point

Further questions specific to Scenario 2 include:

1. Why does the Trust have this policy?

2. What is the evidence to suggest that women with low haemoglobin levels should give birth in hospital?
3. What action can Catherine take to increase her haemoglobin in the next 10 weeks?
4. What would happen if Catherine's haemoglobin was still low at term?
5. How would you support her as her community midwife?

Conclusion

This overview of the routine blood tests offered to pregnant women has highlighted the midwife's role as 'font of all knowledge'. However, the midwife working within a multi-professional team can access the knowledge of specialists when an abnormality or unusual result is reported. Pregnant women are exposed to a range of tests and decisions to make. As advocates for women, midwives must continue to investigate the value of additional tests and treatments, as more become available.

Resources

Food standards agency: http://www. food.gov.uk/.

National Institute for Health and Clinical Excellence (NICE): http://www.nice. org.uk/.

National library for health: http://www.library.nhs.uk/screening/.

National screening committee: http://www.nsc.nhs.uk/.

National study of HIV in pregnancy: http://www.nshpc.ucl.ac.uk/.

Royal College of Obstetricians and Gynaecologists. Management of HIV in pregnancy. Guideline 39: http://www.rcog.org.uk/resources/Public/pdf/RCOG_Guideline_39_low.pdf.

References

Advisory Committee on Immunization Practices: Revised ACIP recommendation for avoiding pregnancy after receiving a rubella-containing vaccine, *MMWR – Morbidity and Mortality Weekly Report* 50:1117, 2001.

Barrett J, Whittaker P, Williams J, et al: Absorption of non-haem iron from food during normal pregnancy, *British Medical Journal* 309:79–82, 1994.

Best JM, O'Shea S, Tipples G, et al: Interpretation of rubella serology in pregnancy – pitfalls and problems, *British Medical Journal* 32S:147–148, 2002.

Bewley C: Medical disorders of pregnancy. In Henderson C, Mayes MS, editors: *Midwifery. A text book for midwives*, ed 13, Edinburgh, 2004, Baillière Tindall.

Chamberlain G, Morgan M: *ABC of antenatal care*, ed 4, London, 2002, BMJ Books.

Coggins J: Iron deficiency anaemia: a complication of pregnancy or a foregone conclusion? A midwife's view, *MIDIRS Midwifery Digest* 11(4):469–474, 2001.

Connor EM, Sperling RS, Gelber R, et al: Reduction of maternal–infant transmission of human immunodeficiency virus type 1 with zidovudine treatment. Pediatric AIDS Clinical Trials Group Protocol 076 Study Group, *New England Journal of Medicine* 331:1173–1180, 1994.

Crowther CA: Anti-D administration in pregnancy for preventing Rhesus alloimmunisation, *Cochrane Review, Cochrane Library*, Issue 4, 2002. Accessed 9/11/02.

Enkin M, Keirse MJNC, Neilson J, et al: *A guide to effective care in pregnancy and childbirth*, ed 3, Oxford, 2000, Oxford University Press.

Hull D, Johnston Dl: *Essential paediatrics*, ed 3, Edinburgh, 1993, Churchill Livingstone.

Jordan S: *Pharmacology for midwives – the evidence base for safe practice*, Basingstoke, 2002, Palgrave.

Luckmann J, Sorensen KC: *Medical and surgical nursing: a psychophysiologic approach*, Philadelphia, 1980, WE Saunders.

McSweeney E, Kirkham J, Vinall P, et al: An audit of anti-D sensitisation in Yorkshire, *British Journal of Obsterics and Gynaecology* 105(10):1091–1094, 1998.

National Health Service Executive: Screening of pregnant women for hepatitis B and immunisation of babies at risk. *Health Service Circular* 1998/127, 1998.

National Institute for Health and Clinical Excellence (NICE): *Technology

Appraisal Guidance No 41. Guidance on the use of routine antenatal anti-D prophylaxis for RhD-negative women, London, 2002, NHS.

National Institute for Health and Clinical Excellence (NICE): *Antenatal care: routine care for the healthy pregnant woman: Clinical guideline 62*, London, 2008, National Collaborating Centre for Women's and Children's Health.

National Screening Committee: UK National Screening Committee's Policy Positions November 2007. Online. Available http://www.nsc.nhs.uk/pdfs/Policy%20Position%20Chart%20Nov%2007.pdf. April 27, 2008.

National Study of HIV in Pregnancy & Childhood (NSHPC): Perinatal transmission of HIV in England 2002–2005, NSHPC, 2007. Online. Available http://www.nshpc.ucl.ac.uk/Audit/Vertical_Transmission_Executive_SummaryOctober_2007.pdf. April 27, 2008

NHS immunisation information: Protecting women against rubella: switch from rubella vaccine to MMR, 2007. Online. Available http://www.immunisation.nhs.uk/Library/News/Protecting_Women_Against_Rubella_Switch_From_Rubella_Vaccine_To_MMR April 26, 2008.

Public Health Laboratory Service, DHSS & PS, Scottish ISD D 5 Collaborative Group: *Sexually transmitted infections in the UK: new episodes seen at Genitourinary Medicine Clinics, 1995–2000*, London, 2001, PHLS.

Reveiz L, Gyte GML, Cuervo LG: Treatments for iron-deficiency anaemia in pregnancy, *Cochrane Database of Systematic Reviews 2001 (updated 2007)* 2(CD003094), 2007.

Royal College of Midwives: *Position Paper 9a. Hepatitis B: a serious hazard*, London, 1999, RCM.

Royal College of Midwives: Anti-D prophylaxis for Rh negative women in pregnancy [letter] 29/01/02. http://www.rcm.org.uk November 9, 2002.

Royal College of Midwives/Department of Health Joint Press Release: *HIV testing in pregnancy – helping women choose*, London, 1999, RCM/DoH.

Royal College of Obstetricians and Gynaecologists: Use of anti-D immunoglobulin for Rh prophylaxis. Guideline 22, 2002. Online. Available http://www.rcog.org.uk/index.asp?PageID=1972 April 27, 2008.

Royal College of Obstetricians and Gynaecologists: Management of HIV in pregnancy. Guideline 39, 2004. Online. Available http://www.rcog.org.uk/resources/Public/pdf/RCOG_Guideline_39_low.pdf November 18, 2008.

Shuttleworth A, editor: *Nursing Times diagnostic procedures*, London, 2002, Emap Healthcare.

Stables D, Rankin J: *Physiology in childbearing with anatomy and related biosciences*, Edinburgh, 2005, Elsevier.

Steer P, Alam MA, Wadsworth J, et al: Relation between maternal haemoglobin concentration and birth weight in different ethnic groups, *British Medical Journal* 310(6978):489–491, 1995.

Stephansson O, Dickman PW, Johansson A, et al: Maternal hemoglobin concentration during pregnancy and risk of stillbirth, *Journal of American Medical Association* 284(20):22–29, 2000.

Symonds E, Symonds I: *Essential obstetrics and gynaecology*, ed 4, Edinburgh, 2004, Churchill Livingstone.

UK Blood Transfusion and Tissue Transplantation Service (Version 4): Handbook of transfusion medicine, 2007a. Online. Available http://www. transfusionguidelines.org.uk/index. aspx?Publication=HTM&Section=9 April 26, 2008.

UK Blood Transfusion and Tissue Transplantation Service: Guidelines for the Blood Transfusion Services in the UK, 2007b. http://www. transfusionguidelines.org.uk/index. aspx?pageid=666&section=25&public ation=RB April 26, 2008.

Antenatal screening for fetal abnormality

Trigger scenario

Joanna is now 32 weeks pregnant. She is feeling very well and finding that now her energy has returned, she is really enjoying being pregnant. She still proudly shows her precious scan picture to interested friends and takes the occasional glance at herself during quiet moments. Joanna has a cousin, Susan, who has Down's syndrome. Susan is a happy and loving child who has brought a lot of joy, as well as heartache, to the extended family. Although Joanna has no delusions about the hard work and continuing care that her cousin requires, she would not herself contemplate terminating a pregnancy if her baby had the condition.

Introduction

Antenatal screening for fetal abnormality is an integral part of routine antenatal care. It is often assumed that women will want to take up this service, just as they would have their urine tested or blood pressure checked. However, what has become routine practice for midwives can have far reaching implications for women. This aspect of antenatal care requires the midwife to be particularly receptive to the cues that women give her and to respect the choices they make. This chapter focuses on antenatal screening for Down's syndrome to illustrate some of the principles that are relevant to screening generally. Tests used for the diagnosis of congenital conditions are summarized, as women need to know what a positive screening test result might lead to.

What is screening?

The terms 'screening' and 'testing' are often used synonymously. However, they are distinctly different and it is important that the midwife is able to convey this difference to women.

Screening is a health service in which members of a defined population, who do not necessarily perceive they are at risk of a disease or its complications, are asked a question or offered a test, to identify those individuals who are more likely to be helped than harmed by further tests or treatment.

(**National Screening Committee 2008a**)

A population is screened to identify people who would benefit from further investigation; that is, those who have a higher risk of the condition being screened for. However, when resources are scarce or when the test itself may potentially cause harm, screening is often limited to a sub-section of a population already deemed to be at higher risk than the rest. As Green & Statham (1993:124) succinctly state, 'if we had cheap, accurate, risk-free diagnostic tests, we would apply them to everybody.'

When screening identifies an individual who has a 'high risk', diagnostic testing is offered to confirm or exclude the condition. Screening usually precedes diagnostic testing; however, individuals already known to be 'high risk' may opt straight for testing if it is offered. The aim of diagnostic testing is to identify if the condition is present and, in the case of antenatal diagnosis for Down's syndrome, to offer the woman the options of continuing with her pregnancy or having a termination.

False positive and negative

Screening is not diagnostic, and it is important that the midwife understands what is meant by a positive or negative screening result. Some results will be positive, that is, fall into an at-risk group, the range of which has previously been determined. However, not all of the cases that fall into that group will have the condition, and they are termed 'false positives'; a result that indicates there is a problem when there is not one.

Some results will be negative; that is, they fall outside of the previously determined at-risk range. However, not all of these cases will be free of the condition being screened for, and these are termed 'false negatives'; a result that indicates there is not a problem, when there is.

These are important considerations, particularly where positive screening may lead to invasive testing in order to confirm the presence or absence of the condition, as is the case with antenatal screening for Down's syndrome. An ideal screening test would be sufficiently sensitive to detect a high proportion of those at risk, without subjecting a large number of people to unnecessary diagnostic testing. The national programme for Down's syndrome screening has a target to detect more than 75% of cases and for a false positive rate of less than 3% (National Screening Committee (NSC) 2007a).

The screening test should meet the following criteria stated by the NSC (2003):

1. There should be a simple, safe, precise and validated screening test
2. The distribution of test values in the target population should be known and a suitable cut-off level defined and agreed
3. The test should be acceptable to the population
4. There should be an agreed policy on the further diagnostic investigation of individuals with a positive test result and the choices available to those people.

Following wide consultation, standards have been developed and agreed by the NSC (2007c), that reflect both generic issues related to antenatal screening and those specific to Down's syndrome. Those relating to antenatal screening tests include policy arrangements, clinical arrangements, education and training for staff: information and support for women and their partners and audit and monitoring processes. Those specific to Down's syndrome comprise: audit and monitoring for Down's syndrome, laboratory standards for Down's syndrome serum screening and ultrasound standards for Down's syndrome screening.

Screening for Down's syndrome

The incidence of Down's syndrome is 1 in 800 births in the general population. This increases with advancing maternal age, from 1 in 1500 births at age 20, to 1 in 280 births at 36 years and 1 in 30 at age 44 (Fetal Anomaly Screening Programme 2007). As the age at which women have their babies increases, finding accurate and acceptable means of screening for Down's syndrome continues to be a relevant issue.

Down's syndrome could potentially occur in any pregnancy. However, women over 35 years of age are particularly at risk of carrying a baby with Down's syndrome and thus maternal age has been a long-standing screening test for this condition. Such 'at-risk' women are often given the option of diagnostic testing, although maternal age as a screening test has limited sensitivity, as approximately 70% of cases of Down's syndrome occur with women under the age of 36 years (Mutton et al 1998). Because of this, and the introduction of new screening tests, screening for Down's syndrome is now offered to all women in early pregnancy (NICE 2008). Screening tests used to identify women at risk of carrying a baby with Down's syndrome include serum screening and ultrasound.

Current provision of screening for Down's syndrome is variable across the UK. A retrospective study, exploring the outcome of 155 501 births over the period 1994–1999, highlighted the variation in screening policies between eight district general hospitals in one health region (Wellesley et al 2002). Screening methods included some or all of the following: maternal age, serum screening, ultrasound scans for nuchal thickness, anomaly and gestational age. Only two hospitals had the same screening policy, and no significant advantage was found for any particular policy, although detection rates ranged form 48% to 58%. Following a survey of consultant obstetricians' attitudes towards screening for Down's syndrome, Green (1994) reported that some obstetricians mentioned the need for a national policy. Such national guidance is now available (NICE 2008) and aims to minimize conflicting information and disparity, through the promotion of clinical practice based on the available evidence. Each Trust should employ a Screening Coordinator to facilitate the implementation of evidence-based policy and guidance (NSC 2007a).

What is serum screening?

Serum screening for Down's syndrome uses a maternal venous blood sample taken by the midwife or phlebotomist. The woman must have had detailed information on which to base her decision to consent to the test. There is a range of serum tests available (Table 8.1). However, following an extensive review of the literature, the National Institute for Health and Clinical Excellence recommends that women who request antenatal screening for Down's syndrome are offered the 'combined test' between 11 weeks 0 days and 13 weeks 6 days (NICE 2008). If the pregnancy is further

advanced, or the nuchal translucency cannot be measured, women should be offered either the 'triple' or 'quadruple' serum screening test, between 15 weeks 0 days and 20 weeks 0 days.

Measurement of markers (Table 8.1) detected in maternal serum is combined with maternal and gestational age, in the calculation of individual risk. Adjustments are made according to maternal weight, so this must be recorded when the test is taken. It has been established that other maternal characteristics, such as ethnic origin, conception via in vitro fertilization and smoking can influence the levels of serum markers in the blood (Kagan et al 2008). Agreed standards for antenatal screening state that 'the cut-off level used to define the population at increased risk of a Down's syndrome affected pregnancy must be 1 in 250 at term' (Fetal Anomaly Screening Programme 2007).

Activity

Find out what screening tests for Down's syndrome are available in your locality.

Discover if they are available to all women, or to a particular sub-section of the pregnant population.

Ultrasound screening for Down's syndrome

The use of scanning in the UK is accepted practice. Not only do women expect to have at least one scan during their pregnancy, but they also expect

Table 8.1 Serum markers for Down's syndrome screening in pregnancy

When	Name	Markers
11 weeks–13 weeks 6 days	Combined test	Serum hCG Serum PAPP-A Ultrasound nuchal translucency
15 weeks–20 weeks	Double	Serum hCG Serum uE3
15 weeks–20 weeks	Triple	Serum hCG Serum uE3 Serum AFP
15 weeks–20 weeks	Quadruple	Serum hCG Serum uE3 Serum AFP Serum inhibin A

Pregnancy-associated plasma protein A (PAPP-A) Beta-human chorionic gonadotrophin (hCG) Unconjugated oestriol (uE3) Alpha feto protein (AFP)

that they will be able to purchase a picture of their unborn baby and in some cases be informed of the baby's sex. Seeing the baby on screen helps make the pregnancy seem more real, for both the woman and her partner (Santalaahti & Hemminiki 1998).

The sensitivity of the scan performed will depend on the resolution of the equipment used, the skill of the ultrasonographer, the gestation and the position of the baby.

From a clinical point of view, the use of routine scanning to date the pregnancy has been justified over the use of last menstrual period (LMP) because it has been shown to reduce the number of inductions for post-maturity (Hogberg & Larsson 1997). Estimation of gestational age by ultrasound rather than on menstrual history also improves the accuracy of serum screening tests

(Brennand & Cameron 2001). In 2002 the Royal College of Obstetricians and Gynaecologists (RCOG 2002) recommended that all women be offered at least one scan to confirm gestational age, preferably followed by an anomaly scan at around 20 weeks' gestation. National guidance recommends that women have a dating scan after 10 weeks and a fetal anomaly scan between 18 and 20 weeks plus 6 days.

A systematic review of women's views of ultrasound scanning during pregnancy indicates that women often lack information regarding the purpose of the scan (Garcia et al 2002). Women were often ignorant that one aim of scanning was to look for markers associated with Down's syndrome. Others assumed that the scan was compulsory and some had unrealistic expectations that the scan confirmed normality.

Nuchal translucency thickness

The fluid that collects behind the neck of the fetus is increased in those who have an abnormality. It can be detected by ultrasound scan and measured; only 10% with a measurement of 6 mm or more will be normal (Berger 1999).

Snijders et al (1998) reported an 82% detection rate for Down's syndrome through the use of a combination of maternal age and fetal nuchal translucency thickness, measured by ultrasonography between 10 and 14 weeks, to select women who were at risk and hence offered diagnostic testing.

Activity

Consider the criteria for screening tests used by the national Screening Committee (NSC).

Decide how far the current screening programme in your locality fulfils these criteria.

Information for women

The booking history is often the first time that women have the opportunity to discuss the issue of screening for fetal abnormality. However, the information that women receive is sometimes less than informative. Women may access information that is brief and misleading. An Australian study revealed that information stated that screening was to make sure that the pregnancy was progressing well, but gave no information about the limitations or reliability of screening (Searle 1997). The increase in the number of options available also adds to the confusion for prospective parents (Saller & Canick 2008).

A content analysis of 80 leaflets available to women in the UK about serum screening for Down's syndrome (Bryant et al 2001) revealed that one third did not contain any descriptive information about the condition. They concluded that more attention needed to be paid to the tone, content and the needs of the reader. A study of 34 women in South Wales found that half the pregnant women had no knowledge of Down's syndrome (Al-Jader et al 2000). The National Screening Committee now produces a comprehensive booklet that provides detailed information about the conditions that can be screened for and the implications of the tests (NSC 2007a).

Lack of knowledge is not confined to pregnant women. In a survey involving 162 midwives in a large Trust, 41% demonstrated poor knowledge related to Down's syndrome screening and only 39% of the midwives who responded felt confident to counsel women adequately about screening (Samwill 2002). Perceived ability to facilitate informed choice in antenatal screening was also limited in a study conducted by Wray & Maresh (2000) and again echoed in a recent Australian study (Noseworthy & Cooper 2007). Education and training of midwives regarding all aspects of screening is the responsibility of local screening coordinators, in liaison with pre- and post-registration education providers and local Trusts. However, individual midwives must also take responsibility to keep up-to-date with new practices and technologies (NMC 2008). There is a plethora of resources to support midwives in this challenging aspect of their role (Harcombe 2007).

The midwife must be aware that the choices women and their partners make about antenatal screening for fetal abnormality are not solely based on the information they receive in pregnancy. They may have had long-standing views following the experiences of their family and friends. Religious and cultural values will also impact on the course that women take. Knowing that they would never terminate a pregnancy, for whatever reason, will prevent some women from having a screening test. Other women may be against termination but feel that they want to know if their baby has an increased risk of having the condition. Some women will feel strongly that they would want their baby, whatever problems it had. Others might feel that it is wrong to birth a baby that might have a reduced quality of life. That individuals come to a parent partnership with potentially different views also means that they need to find a stance from which they both feel comfortable, and this may take time.

Midwives must also be aware of the impact that their body language has on their interactions with women, and demonstrate to each woman that they are listening (Baston 2002). Stapelton et al (2002) report how women often respond to midwives' apparent busyness

by withholding questions, and that midwives often mistake a woman's silence for lack of interest. Midwives need to make an effort to establish on what basis a woman is making a choice, in order to ensure that she is making a decision based on understanding. It has been shown that providing more information about screening in pregnancy does not increase overall anxiety (Thornton et al 1995). The midwife has an important role in presenting balanced, relevant information in an understandable manner. She must be able to identify and rectify lack of knowledge, whilst acknowledging and addressing her own limitations.

In summary

Before agreeing to have a screening test for Down's syndrome, the woman and her partner need to know:

- What Down's syndrome is
- That the test is not compulsory
- That the midwife will support the woman, whatever choice she makes
- What the test is for and that it is only designed to screen for a particular syndrome
- That it is not a diagnostic test and will only give an indication of individual risk
- What the false positive/negative rate is and what this means
- That they might be offered further tests if they are found to be 'high risk'
- That the diagnosis can only be made following an invasive procedure which has a 1% risk of miscarriage
- How results will be given.

Activity

Make sure you are aware of how women currently receive the results of screening tests where you work.

Think about who is best placed to provide an at-risk result.

Find out what populations are most at risk of haemoglobinopathy.

Haemoglobinopathies

Haemoglobin is a protein that is found in the red blood cells of the blood which carries oxygen around the body. A haemoglobinopathy is a genetic (therefore inherited) abnormality of haemoglobin; in the United Kingdom the most common are sickle cell anaemia and thalassaemia.

Sickle cell anaemia

This is a recessive genetic disorder, therefore both parents need to be carriers (have sickle cell trait) for a person to inherit sickle cell disease. In this condition the affected person has abnormal red blood cells because of an abnormality of the haemoglobin; a form known as Hb-S. During situations where oxygen is scarce, for example during exercise or stress, the red blood cells become 'banana' shaped and clump together. This can lead to small blood vessels becoming blocked which deprives the area of oxygen and causes severe pain; this is known as a sickle cell crisis. There are more than 12 500 people with sickle cell disease

and approximately 240 000 healthy carriers in the UK (National Screening Committee 2008b).

Thalassaemia

This is a term used to describe recessive genetic disorders which result in a reduction in the amount of haemoglobin produced by the body (UK Newborn Screening Programme Centre (UKNSPC) 2007). There are two types of thalassaemia, alpha and beta, depending on the type of globin chains that are too few in number.

In alpha thalassaemia, carriers often have anaemia, with reduced mean corpuscular haemoglobin (MCH) and mean corpuscular volume (MCV) due to the production of insufficient alpha globin chains. If no alpha globin is produced because of no functioning alpha genes, this is incompatible with life (alpha thalassaemia major) (NICE 2008). In beta thalassaemia, if one affected gene is inherited, the person has 3.5% abnormal haemoglobin, is a carrier but does not have the disease (NICE 2008). However, if beta thalassaemia major is inherited, the affected person will have severe anaemia leading to death if untreated. Individuals can survive if they have regular blood transfusions or a successful bone marrow transplant. Complications of the disease include: organ failure, skeletal deformity and reduced life expectancy (NICE 2008). There are more than 700 people with thalassaemia disorders and approximately 214 000 healthy carriers in the UK (National Screening Committee 2008b).

Screening for haemoglobinopathies

All pregnant women should be screened for haemoglobinopathy in early pregnancy (NICE 2008). In low prevalence areas (fetal prevalence 1.5 affected cases per 10 000 pregnancies, or less) women should be asked to complete the Family Origin Questionnaire (FOQ) (National Screening Committee 2006). In high prevalence areas (fetal prevalence above 1.5 affected cases per 10 000 pregnancies) or where women in low prevalence areas are identified at risk through the FOQ, women should be offered laboratory screening (high performance liquid chromatography). If the woman is subsequently identified as a carrier of either sickle cell disease or thalassaemia, the father of the baby should also be offered information and counselling, and possible screening (NICE 2008).

Screening for structural abnormalities

All women should be offered ultrasound screening for structural defects between 18 and 20 weeks 6 days (NICE 2008). Having a scan in pregnancy is often anticipated as a positive experience and while it is important not to detract from this opportunity to 'see' their developing baby, women need to be informed that the purpose is to look for abnormalities. They should also know that although this scan is available to all women, that does not mean that they are obliged to have it. The National Screening Committee has produced a comprehensive leaflet about the mid-pregnancy scan (NSC 2007b).

Activity

Find out which structural abnormalities can be identified by ultrasound scan at 20 weeks of pregnancy.

For each of these anomalies, make sure you know the accuracy of this screening test.

Antenatal diagnostic tests

If a woman is found to be at risk of carrying a baby with Down's syndrome, she will be offered diagnostic testing.

Cytogenic techniques

Cytogenetics is the study of chromosomes and the related disease states caused by numerical and structural chromosome abnormalities. The process of identifying the chromosomal make-up of an individual is called karyotyping.

In order to obtain a diagnosis of Down's syndrome, it is necessary to examine the fetal chromosomes in the laboratory. Normally, in a human cell, there are 23 pairs of chromosomes (46 in total). However, in Down's syndrome there is an extra chromosome number 21 (47 in total), hence the term

Trisomy 21 which is used to describe this condition. This process involves identifying the chromosomes and hence requires the fetal cells to be sufficiently grown. New methods for examining chromosomes continue to be developed enabling results to be obtained faster than before. For example, fluorescent in situ hybridization (FISH) is a technique which involves looking at a specific chromosome rather than all of them, and takes about 3 days, thus providing a comparatively quick result (Seres-Santamaria et al 1993). Another method capable of identifying chromosomal abnormalities is quantitative polymerase chain reaction (Q-PCR). Both of these techniques are of limited availability, depending on the facilities and skills available in the local laboratory.

Procedures for obtaining fetal cells include amniocentesis, chorionic villus sampling and cordocentesis.

Before agreeing to diagnostic testing the woman and her partner need to know:

- What the test involves
- That it can detect other chromosomal abnormalities
- That there is a risk of miscarriage or infection
- That the result may take up to 3 weeks
- That occasionally the fetal cells do not grow and a result cannot be given
- How results will be given
- That they would be offered termination of the pregnancy if Down's syndrome was diagnosed.

Amniocentesis

This procedure is usually carried out between 15 and 20 weeks of pregnancy. It involves removal of about 10–20 ml of amniotic fluid from around the fetus and is performed using ultrasound guidance. Fetal cells are cultured, and this can take up to 3 weeks or more. Sometimes, but rarely, the cells fail to grow. There is an associated miscarriage rate of approximately 1% and there is also a small risk of infection, bleeding and premature rupture of the fetal membranes.

Chorionic villus sampling

This procedure involves removal of a sample of villi from the chorion frondosum, either transcervically or through the abdomen, and has the advantage of being performed during the first trimester of pregnancy, usually between 11–13 weeks. Provisional results are usually available within 1 week, as fetal cells do not need to be cultured. There is an associated 2–3% miscarriage rate but because it is performed during the first trimester it is difficult to determine which miscarriages might have occurred naturally.

Cordocentesis

Percutaneous umbilical blood sampling (PUBS) or cordocentesis involves inserting a needle through the woman's abdomen directly into the umbilical artery or vein in order to take a sample of fetal blood. It is performed under ultrasound guidance and carries the risks associated with amniocentesis.

It is not normally attempted before 18 weeks' gestation and is not routinely used for diagnostic purposes in the UK.

Reflection on trigger scenario

Look back on the trigger scenario.

Joanna is now 32 weeks pregnant. She is feeling very well and finding that now her energy has returned, she is really enjoying being pregnant. She still proudly shows her precious scan picture to interested friends and takes the occasional glance at herself during quiet moments. Joanna has a cousin, Susan, who has Down's syndrome. Susan is a happy and loving child who has brought a lot of joy, as well as heartache, to the extended family. Although Joanna has no delusions about the hard work and continuing care that her cousin requires, she would not herself contemplate terminating a pregnancy if her baby had the condition.

Now that you are familiar with the issues regarding antenatal screening for fetal abnormality you should have insight into how the scenario relates to current midwfery practice. The jigsaw model will now be used to explore the trigger scenario in more depth.

Effective communication

Communication between the midwife and expectant parents is paramount if the midwife is to ensure that they understand the implications of undergoing antenatal screening for fetal abnormality. Questions that arise from the scenario might include: What information did Joanna receive about antenatal screening for fetal abnormality? When did she receive it and in what format? Did Joanna share the information with her partner Louis? Did she understand the information she received? Did she have the opportunity to ask the midwife for clarification about aspects of the screening on offer?

Woman-centred care

Any screening programme, whether locally developed or following national guidelines, must ultimately be tailored to the individual needs of the family expecting the baby. Everyone comes to pregnancy with there own catalogue of hopes and fears and these need to be acknowledged if the pregnancy is to be a positive experience. Questions that arise from the scenario might include: Did the midwife ask Joanna if she had thought about the implications of having a baby with Down's syndrome? Did Joanna talk about her cousin Susan when she discussed screening tests with the midwife? Was there enough time for Joanna to voice her own particular view about having a baby with Down's syndrome? Did Joanna feel any pressure to have a serum screening test?

Using best evidence

When making a potentially life and death decision, the woman should feel that it has been based on the best available evidence. She should feel that the midwife is giving her information based on a sound understanding of the current knowledge base.

Questions that arise from the scenario might include: What resources can the midwife provide for women who are making decisions about antenatal screening? Is there an audit of the process and the outcome of antenatal screening for fetal abnormality? What action has been taken recently to enhance the antenatal screening service that Joanna has accessed?

Professional and legal issues

Before undergoing screening for fetal abnormality it is essential that women are able to give informed consent. This means that information has to be presented in such a way that it is meaningful and makes sense to both the woman and her partner.

Questions that arise from the scenario might include: What aspect of the NMC Code (NMC 2008) are particularly pertinent to gaining informed consent from a woman? What action should be taken by the midwife if a woman declines screening? What is the law around termination of pregnancy for fetal abnormality? Under what circumstances can a midwife perform ultrasonography?

Team working

Screening for fetal abnormality involves a range of professionals each with a valuable and essential role to take, from venepuncture to conveying the result. There is a need for a robust care pathway to ensure that each member of the team takes responsibility for their particular role. Questions that arise from the scenario might include:

Who did Joanna meet in relation to considering antenatal screening for fetal abnormality? How would the fact that Joanna declined the test be viewed by the antenatal screening coordinator? Did Joanna's partner agree with the stance Joanna has taken? How might his attitude have influenced her decision?

Clinical dexterity

The midwife involved in screening for fetal abnormality needs to have developed dexterity in handling a range of clinical scenarios. She needs to be able to give impartial information to women considering screening and also to be able to inform some women that their result has placed them at high risk of having an affected baby. Questions that arise from the scenario might include: What do women expect from their midwife throughout the screening process? Are all midwives adept at breaking bad news? What was Joanna's midwife's reaction to her declining screening?

Models of care

Women access maternity services through a variety of systems. Some go straight to their GP when they discover they are pregnant and others access maternity services by going directly to a midwife. Questions that arise from the scenario might include: At what point was Joanna given information to help her make the right choice for her individual circumstances? Did she think about these issues before she had even become pregnant? What facts might make a woman change her mind?

Does the profession of the person who counsels her regarding the tests available make a difference to her decision?

Safe environment

When a woman decides to have or to decline a screening test, she needs to feel secure in the decision she has made. She needs to have gone through a process whereby the decision is as clear and unambiguous as possible, having had the opportunity to explore the implications thoroughly. Questions that arise from the scenario might include: What organizational factors could compromise the safety of a woman's decision regarding antenatal screening? What emotional, social and cultural factors might impact on Joanna's decision to decline screening? What support will Joanna have if she births a baby with Down's syndrome?

Promotes health

The midwife has a key role to play in facilitating positive physical and emotional wellbeing for the woman and her family throughout the childbirth continuum. The midwife must therefore respect the woman's autonomy and agency to make decisions that are right for her. Questions that arise from the scenario might include: How can the midwife demonstrate her respect for Joanna and support her in her choices? What resources can the midwife provide for women who are contemplating pregnancy and wanting to adopt a healthy lifestyle in preparation?

Further scenarios

The following scenarios enable you to consider how specific situations influence the care the midwife provides. Use the jigsaw model to explore the issues raised in the scenario.

Scenario 1

Claire is 6 weeks pregnant with her first baby. She has just been to see her general practitioner who asked her if she was taking folic acid. When Claire said that she was not, the GP told her to start taking it as it might reduce her chances of having a baby with spina bifida.

Practice point

Further questions specific to Scenario 1 include:

1. When does the neural tube develop and close?
2. What is the recommended dose of folic acid in pregnancy?
3. Which women are at increased risk of having a baby with a neural tube defect?
4. Which foods are naturally rich in folic acid?
5. Which foods are fortified with folic acid?
6. What are the physical sequelae for a child with spina bifida?

Scenario 2

Gemma was born in the United Kingdom and both her parents are African Caribbean. Two months ago she went on holiday with her friends to Morocco and met a local man, Theo, whom she began dating. They were inseparable all holiday and she has kept in touch with him through email and texting ever since. Last week she was delighted to find out that she is pregnant with his baby.

Practice point

Further questions specific to Scenario 2 include:

1. Which haemoglobinopathies is Gemma's baby at risk of inheriting?
2. How would this risk be verified at the booking appointment?
3. Where should Gemma be referred for expert counselling?

4. Which professionals provide genetic counselling?
5. How can Gemma involve Theo in the counselling process?

Conclusion

Antenatal screening and diagnosis for fetal abnormality is a complex issue. Midwives are required to continually update their knowledge and skills. This aspect of antenatal care presents many challenges as new programmes and technologies come into the arena and midwives need to work closely with the multi-professional team to provide a seamless service for antenatal women.

Resources

Antenatal results and choices: http://www.arc-uk.org/.

Down's syndrome screening education and training pack: http://www.screening.nhs.uk/cpd/downs.htm.

Family origin questionnaire screening for haemoglobinopathy: http://phs.kcl.ac.uk/haemscreening/Documents/F_Origin_Questionnaire.pdf.

Interviews with women and couples to find out their experiences of

antenatal screening: www.dipex.org/antenatalscreening.

National Screening Committee Induction information for new staff about screening programmes: http://www.screening.nhs.uk/cpd/induction.htm.

NHS Sickle Cell & Thalassaemia Screening Programme: http://www.sickleandthal.org.uk/.

UK Newborn Screening Programme Centre Glossary of terms: http://www.ich.ucl.ac.uk/newborn/glossary/index.htm.

References

Al-Jader LN, Parry-Langdon N, Smith RJ: Survey of attitudes of pregnant women towards Down's syndrome screening, *Prenatal Diagnosis* 20(10):23–29, 2000.

Baston H: Midwifery basics. Antenatal care – the booking history, *The Practising Midwife* 5(10):26–30, 2002.

Berger A: What is fetal nuchal translucency? *British Medical Journal* 318(7176):85, 1999.

Brennand JE, Cameron AD: Current methods of screening for Down's syndrome, Reprinted in MIDIRS Midwifery Digest 12(2):183–188, *The Obstetrician and Gynecologist* 3(4): 191–197, 2001.

Bryant LD, Murray J, Green JM, et al: Descriptive information about Down's syndrome: a content analysis of serum screening leaflets, *Prenatal Diagnosis* 21(12):1057–1063, 2001.

Fetal Anomaly Screening Programme: Screening information, 2007. Online. Available http://nscfa.web.its. manchester.ac.uk/ April 28, 2008.

Garcia J, Bricker L, Henderson J, et al: Women's views of pregnancy ultrasound: a systematic review, *Birth* 29(4):225–249, 2002.

Green JM: Serum screening for Down's syndrome: experiences of obstetricians in England and Wales, *British Medical Journal* 309:769–772, 1994.

Green I, Statham H: Testing for fetal abnormality in routine antenatal care, *Midwifery* 9:124–135, 1993.

Harcombe: Supporting midwives in screening, *Midwives* 10(1):28–30, 2007.

Hogberg U, Larsson N: Early dating by ultrasound and perinatal outcome: a cohort study, *Acta Obstetrica et Gynecologica Scandinavica* 76(10): 907–912, 1997.

Kagan K, Wright D, Spencer K, et al: First-trimester screening for trisomy 21 by free beta-human chorionic gonadotrophin and pregnancy associated plasma protein-A: impact of maternal and pregnancy characteristics, *Ultrasound in Obstetrics and Gynecology* 31(5):493–502, 2008.

Mutton D, Ide RG, Alberman E: Trends in prenatal screening for diagnosis of Down's syndrome: England and Wales, 1987–97, *British Medical Journal* 317:922–923, 1998.

National Institute for Health and Clinical Excellence (NICE): *Antenatal care: routine care for the healthy pregnant woman. Clinical Guideline 62*, London, 2008, National Collaborating Centre for Women's and Children's Health.

National Screening Committee: Criteria for appraising the viability, effectiveness and appropriateness of a screening programme, 2003. Online. Available http://www.nsc.nhs.uk/uk_nsc/uk_nsc_ ind.htm. April 28, 2008.

National Screening Committee: National Screening Committee policy- sickle cell and thalassaemia screening (in pregnancy), 2006. Online. Available http://www.library.nhs.uk/screening/ ViewResource.aspx?resID=32452&tabI D=288&catID=8208 April 27, 2008.

National Screening Committee: *Screening tests for you and your baby*, Oxford, 2007a, NSC.

National Screening Committee: *Having a mid-pregnancy ultrasound scan?* Exeter, 2007b, NSC.

National Screening Committee: *Antenatal screening – working standards for Down's syndrome screening. National*

Down's Syndrome Screening Programme for England, Exeter, 2007c, NSC.

National Screening Committee: National Screening Committee Induction information for new staff about screening programmes, 2008a. Online. Available http://www.screening.nhs.uk/cpd/induction.htm. April 28, 2008.

National Screening Committee: Glossary for UK national screening programmes, 2008b. Online. Available http://www.nsc.nhs.uk/glossary/glossary_ind.htm. April 28, 2008.

Nursing and Midwifery Council (NMC): *The code. Standards of conduct, performance and ethics for nurses and midwives*, London, 2008, NMC.

Noseworthy D, Cooper M: Screening in the childbearing year: midwives' scientific knowledge and its use in decision making, *Canadian Journal of Midwifery Research and Practice* 6(2):33–40, 2007.

Royal College of Obstetricians and Gynaecologists: *Clinical standards – advice on planning the service in obstetrics and gynaecology*, London, 2002, RCOG Press.

Saller D, Canick J: Current methods of prenatal screening for Down syndrome and other fetal abnormalities, *Clinical Obstetrics and Gynecology* 51(1):24–36, 2008.

Samwill L: Midwives' knowledge of Down's syndrome screening, *Midwifery* 10(4):247–250, 2002.

Santalaahti P, Hemminiki E: On what grounds do women participate in prenatal screening? *Prenatal Diagnosis* 18(2):153–165, 1998.

Searle J: Routine antenatal screening: not a case of informed choice, *Australian and New Zealand Journal of Public Health* 21(3):268–274, 1997.

Seres-Santamaria A, Catal V, Cuatrecasas E, et al: Fluorescent in-situ hybridisation and Down's syndrome, *The Lancet* 341(8859):1544, 1993.

Snijders R, Noble P, Sebire N, et al: UK multicentre project on assessment of risk of trisomy 21 by maternal age and fetal nuchal translucency thickness at 10–14 weeks of gestation, *The Lancet* 352(9125):343–346, 1998.

Stapelton H, Kirkham M, Curtis P, et al: Silence and time in antenatal care, *British Journal of Midwifery* 10(6): 393–396, 2002.

Thornton I, Hewison I, Lilford RI, et al: A randomised trial of three methods of giving information about prenatal testing, *British Medical Journal* 311:1127–1130, 1995.

UK Newborn Screening Programme Centre: Glossary of terms, 2007. Online. Available http://www.ich.ucl.ac.uk/newborn/glossary/index.htm. April 27, 2008.

Wellesley D, Boyle T, Barber I, et al: Retrospective audit of different antenatal screening policies for Down's syndrome in eight district general hospitals in one health region, *British Medical Journal* 325(7354):15, 2002.

Wray I, Maresh M: Midwives, obstetricians and prenatal screening, *British Journal of Midwifery* 8(1): 31–35, 2000.

Monitoring fetal wellbeing during routine antenatal care

Trigger scenario

Joanna is now 36 weeks into her pregnancy and feeling well but tired. The baby seems to be most active at night when she is trying to sleep – she doesn't seem to notice the movements during the day. Jo has developed some stretch marks at the top of her legs and is hoping that they will not appear on her tummy as she likes wearing low-waisted jeans. Her partner has not yet heard the baby's heartbeat and is hoping to take time off work to go with Jo for her next antenatal appointment.

Introduction

A significant aspect of the midwife's role in the antenatal period is to monitor the health of the woman and of her unborn child. This chapter focuses on the role of the midwife in monitoring the wellbeing of the developing fetus during routine antenatal care. As antenatal care usually takes place within the community setting in the United Kingdom this chapter will concentrate on the antenatal examination within this arena. The skill of abdominal palpation with regard to monitoring growth, activity and the fetal heart rate, will be described.

Background

Consideration for the wellbeing of the fetus should not be taken in isolation from the wellbeing of the mother, as they are both intrinsically interlinked. Pregnancy is a time of change for women and their families and the relationship she has with her unborn baby is complex. Many fear that the wellbeing of their baby may have been inadvertently compromised. In a large questionnaire-based survey it was shown that women commonly feared there was something wrong with their babies, particularly at the beginning and end of pregnancy (Statham et al 1997). Part of a midwife's role is to enhance a woman's wellbeing through reassurance that her baby is growing and developing at an appropriate rate, through appropriate monitoring techniques (NMC 2004).

National guidance

The NICE Guidelines for antenatal care (NICE 2008) provide guidance for caring for the woman and her fetus. They state that midwives should always treat women:

with kindness, respect and dignity... The views, beliefs and values of the woman, her partner and her family in relation to her care and that of her baby should be sought and respected at all times... Women should have the opportunity to make informed decisions about their care and treatment, in partnership with their healthcare professionals

(NICE 2008:37)

The guidelines state that the number of appointments required: 'in order to successfully monitor the baby should be dependent on the needs of the mother and baby.' (NICE 2008:72). This means that the midwife should provide a flexible approach to care and using her professional judgment over the woman's and baby's needs.

Professional guidance

In the midwives rules of practice (NMC 2004) it states that the needs of the woman or baby should be the 'primary focus'. In the EU activities of a midwife, one of the roles is:

Activity

Access the NICE antenatal guideline: http://www.nice.org.uk/guidance/index.jsp?action=download&o=40145 and look at section 4:7 What should happen at antenatal appointments?: the suggested patterns of care for nuilliparous and multiparous women.
  Access http://www.nice.org.uk/guidance/index.jsp?action=download&o=40115 and look at section 1.10 on Fetal growth and wellbeing. Consider the midwife's role in monitoring the growth of the baby.

To diagnose pregnancies and monitor normal pregnancies; to carry out examinations necessary for the monitoring of the development of normal pregnancies.

(NMC 2004)

Students are expected to learn skills of communication in the antenatal period, as well as to 'assess and monitor women holistically' through the whole pregnancy continuum 'through the use of a range of assessment methods and reach valid, reliable and comprehensive conclusions', further: 'to carry out examinations necessary for the monitoring of the development of normal pregnancies.' (NMC 2009)

Monitoring fetal wellbeing

Assessing fetal growth

During the antenatal examination, the midwife uses a range of methods to assess fetal growth, including sensitive use of discussion, palpation and measurement.

Discussion with the woman

Probably the most important gauge of fetal growth is the woman's own estimation. She is the one who is living with her growing uterus and able to note the impact of her changing shape on her daily life. She may be finding it more difficult to bend over and pick dropped items from the floor as fundal height increases. Alternatively, earlier in pregnancy she might be concerned that she has not yet needed to buy any maternity clothes. A simple question such as, 'How do you think your baby has grown since we last met?' provides an opportunity for her to voice any concerns.

Women may worry about the growth of their baby at both ends of the scale. Fear that it is growing rapidly may raise doubts about her ability to have a vaginal birth. Worry that the baby is too small may cause concern about its development and health. Concern about fetal growth can also change over time, with women worrying that they are not growing enough in early pregnancy and then too much as pregnancy advances and thoughts of the birth become more prominent.

Verbal consent to palpate the woman's abdomen should be gained at each examination. Although it will not be appropriate to launch into a full-blown explanation about what you are going to do each time you meet, if you have never met the woman before, or it is the first time she has attended the clinic, she needs to know what the palpation

will involve. As a midwife, you will develop your own way of asking permission to undertake procedures, but avoid the use of statements such as, 'I'm just going to…' or 'Just pop up on the couch'. Consent should not be assumed, and such language can come across as condescending. Where any language difficulties are anticipated, an interpreter should be used.

Having ensured that the woman does not have a full bladder, that she understands what you aim to do and that she agrees to it, ask her to sit on the couch. She should be asked to undo or loosen her clothing before you lower the headrest, so that she can see what she is doing. The headrest should not be totally flat. Her legs should be covered with a modesty sheet and her arms by her side. The equipment required for palpation is listed in Box 9.1.

Inspection

The first observation that the midwife makes, before she lays her hands on the woman, is to inspect the abdomen for shape, scars, skin and size (the four S's):

Shape

The uterus of the primigravida is ovoid in shape compared with the more rounded shape of multigravida. The abdomen should be inspected for curves and dips that might give clues regarding the fetal position. If the fetus has adopted an anterior position it may be possible to detect the curve of the fetal back. A fetus in the posterior position might give the abdomen a dip

Box 9.1 Equipment required for abdominal palpation

• **Pinard's stethoscope** **Rationale** To locate the fetal heart	• **Tissues** **Rationale** To remove excess jelly from the woman's abdomen
• **Doppler** **Rationale** To enable the woman/partner/children to hear the fetal heart	• **Disposable or washable tape measure** **Rationale** To measure the symphysis–fundal height tape measure
• **Aqueous jelly** **Rationale** To facilitate contact with the Doppler transducer and maternal abdomen	• **Modesty sheet** **Rationale** To cover woman's legs

or hollow (best observed by looking at the abdomen at eye level).

Scars

Abdominal scars should be noted and should correspond with the 'previous medical history' taken at the booking visit. Women may need reassurance that a scar will not burst open, but that the skin will gradually stretch to accommodate the growing fetus.

Activity

List three indications for abdominal surgery.

For each one, note down where you would expect to find the scar.

Think about why it is important that scars are noted during abdominal palpation.

Skin

A line of pigmentation (linea nigra) may be noted extending centrally from the symphysis pubis to the umbilicus. The skin might appear tight and shiny

if there is an excess of amniotic fluid (polyhydramnios), and further clinical signs should be considered to identify a potential case requiring referral to a medical practitioner (NMC 2004). Of considerable distress to some women is the development of stretch marks (striae gravidarum). These appear as red lines which eventually fade to silver after the birth. However, they can be itchy and cause considerable irritation, and the midwife should acknowledge the woman's discomfort, offering practical advice as well as listening to her concerns. There are many preparations available on the market for

Activity

Find out what potential fetal anomalies are associated with polyhydramnios and oligohydramnios.

Make sure you know what the woman might complain of when there is excess amniotic fluid.

Make yourself aware of the clinical significance of acute and/or chronic polyhydramnios.

the 'prevention' and treatment of stretch marks; however the evidence of their benefit is limited and daily massage may be more effective (Young & Jewell 1996). Keeping cool and keeping the skin well moisturized and hydrated may prevent further exacerbation of this condition.

Size

The first estimation of fetal growth is made by the midwife when she observes the abdomen. However, this is only part of the picture and one that can be entirely misleading, depending on the tone of the abdominal musculature, the amount of amniotic fluid, the accumulation of subcutaneous fat and fetal position. Further clinical assessments are required before fetal size can be more accurately judged, although clinical estimation of fetal weight is notoriously inaccurate (Enkin et al 2000).

Palpation

This essential practical skill takes time to develop and, like all skills, improves with practice. The hands of a midwife become her most powerful tools, with which she can convey care as well as detect both maternal and fetal wellbeing.

Before the procedure, the woman should be encouraged to empty her bladder. She might be advised to go to the toilet when she arrives at the antenatal clinic rather than during the consultation, but her comfort should be reassessed prior to the palpation. If she is trying to hold on to a full bladder, her abdominal muscles may be tense and palpation uncomfortable. A full

bladder can significantly affect fundal height (Engstrom et al 1989) and lead to undue concern about fetal growth.

Maintaining privacy and dignity throughout the palpation is essential. If possible, the examination couch should be arranged so that the woman's feet are away from the door and that her left-hand side (if the midwife is right-handed) is against a wall. There should be a fold-out step to enable the woman to reach the couch with ease and an adjustable headrest should be made use of. A sheet should be used to cover the woman's legs, even if she still has trousers on. This conveys the message that you understand that she is exposing her body and that you will continue to take steps to minimize this exposure.

The woman must feel safe and the focus of the midwife's attention at all times. Of course, this should be so during all points of contact between the woman and the midwife, but it is especially important when the woman is lying down and the midwife is standing up. This physical dominance must not be transferred into a superiority that prevents or spoils meaningful communication.

Estimation of gestational age

The next part of the palpation involves estimation of gestational age and size. The midwife, usually standing with the woman's head to her left, uses her warm, clean hands to locate the uterine fundus. First, she applies the pads of the fingers of the left hand to the abdomen, just below the woman's xiphisternum. Using a gentle pressing movement, the midwife works her way down the abdomen until she feels the resistance of the fundus.

The midwife uses three landmarks when assessing gestational age by palpation: the xiphisternum, the umbilicus and the symphysis pubis. She estimates that, at approximately 12 weeks of pregnancy, the fundus is palpable above the symphysis pubis. It rises approximately a centimetre each week thereafter, being between the pubis and the umbilicus at 16 weeks and at the umbilicus by about 22–24 weeks. By 32 weeks the fundus is midway between the umbilicus and xiphisternum. At 36 weeks the gravid uterus has reached the xiphisternum and in subsequent weeks, as the presenting part enters the pelvis, the fundal height descends slightly ('lightening'). The overall size of the uterus must be taken into account, however, as fundal height will vary depending on the fetal lie.

The ability to assess gestational age is a midwifery skill that develops with experience. Continuity of care in the community will aid the detection of babies whose growth begins to deviate from normal parameters. Fetal growth restriction is associated with poor neonatal outcome (Berghella 2007). In an attempt to employ a more 'objective' method of monitoring fetal size, physical measurement has been advocated. Conveniently, average fetal growth is about 1 centimetre (cm) per week. This has enabled midwives and obstetricians to use the tape measure to determine fetal growth. The tape is held at the fundus and extended to the symphysis pubis (from the variable to the fixed point). For a

more objective measurement, it should be held so that the centimetre side is applied to the woman's abdomen and more than one measurement taken. This practice has been part of UK national guidance since 2003 (NICE) and it remains a recommendation that fundal height is measured at each examination after 24 weeks' gestation (NICE 2008:37).

Activity

Find out the local policy for measurement of fundal height in your Trust.

Discover what action should be taken if the fundal height is smaller or larger than expected for the gestation.

However, this method of estimating fetal growth has been critisized for a range of reasons, including uncertainty regarding where to take the measurement from and to (Engstrom & Sittler 1993), discrepancies between examiners (Engstrom et al 1993a) and differences in measurements due to maternal position (Engstrom et al 1993b). Neilson (1998), in a systematic review of the controlled trials on this issue, concluded that there is insufficient evidence to evaluate the use of symphysis–fundal height measurement in pregnancy, but that it would be unwise to abandon its use unless a large trial suggests that it is unhelpful.

Gardosi & Francis (1999) evaluated the use of customized charts (adjusted for maternal height, weight in early pregnancy, parity and ethnic origin) for plotting serial measurement of fundal height. They found that the use of such charts by community midwives led to an increase in the detection of small for gestational age babies (48% in the study group compared with 29% of controls) and large for gestational age babies (46% in the study group compared with 24% of controls). McGeown (2001) provides a useful overview of the chart used. The use of this tool has been debated at length, for example, Zhang et al (2007). Their use has not been recommended by NICE for routine use and this has been contested by the Perinatal Institute who strongly advocate their value (Perinatal Institute 2008).

Fundal, lateral and pelvic palpation

The remainder of the palpation focuses on determining the lie, presentation and position of the fetus. The student midwife is encouraged to adopt a systematic approach to this technique and to practise translating her findings into professional language. However she must not lose sight of the fact that the woman will need an ongoing commentary of what the midwife is feeling, and the woman should be encouraged to contribute to the detective work. Ascertaining the position and presentation of the baby is recommended at 36 weeks of pregnancy, so that babies in breech presentation can be identified and women offered external cephalic version (NICE 2008).

For a brief summary of abdominal palpation, see Box 9.2.

Fetal movements

During the palpation, the midwife will involve the woman by asking her where she feels most of her movements. In combination with what she is feeling, this information will help the midwife to deduce the fetal position. In addition, she will ask the woman about the fetus's general activity and address any concerns that the woman might have. There is no evidence to suggest that routine counting of fetal movements has any beneficial outcome (Mangesi & Hofmeyr 2007) and is not therefore recommended routinely (NICE 2008:37). As pregnancy advances there is less room for the baby to move, and movements therefore feel different; the baby should remain active for the whole pregnancy and, indeed, during labour.

Fetal activity is used as a determinant of fetal wellbeing. James (2002) states that 'reduced fetal activity is the only assessment shown to identify fetuses at risk of intrauterine death'. In a prospective study of 752 pregnancies at or over 35 weeks' gestation, Berbey et al (2001) concluded that reduced fetal movements were predictive of abnormal NST, low Apgars, meconium-stained liquor and intrapartum fetal distress.

When a reduction in fetal movements is reported by a pregnant woman, a cardiotocograph (CTG) recording fetal heart rate, fetal movements and uterine

---

Box 9.2 Summary of abdominal palpation

- **FUNDAL PALPATION**

Technique   Place both hands gently around the fundus, using the pads of closed fingers to determine contours of the fetus.

Rationale   To determine the contents of the upper pole of the uterus. To inform pelvic palpation

Findings   The head feels hard and is ballotable. Note the size in relation to fundal height – breech is broader and neck is not distinguishable

- **LATERAL PALPATION**

Technique   Imagine the uterus is half an orange and there are six segments. Facing the woman, keep left hand at the left side of the uterus (her right). Use the pads of the fingers of the right hand to work down the fundus, starting at the most lateral edge, segment 1. Keeping the left hand still, repeat from the top, but moving anteriorly to segment 2. Repeat on segment 3. Now use the right hand to steady the right side of the uterus and repeat for segments 6, 5 and 4

Rationale   To keep the fetus steady to enable the position of the fetal back to be identified. To use a systematic approach to locate the fetal back. To determine the position of the fetus

Findings   The back continues from the breech down. It is distinguishable from the irregular feel of the fetal limbs. Contours can be followed down to the shoulder and neck. Detection of the back at the far sides of uterus (segment 1–2 or 6–5) = lateral position. Location at segment 2–3 or 5–4 = anterior position. Back not easily felt but limbs felt anteriorly = posterior position

- **PELVIC PALPATION**

Technique   Midwife faces woman's feet and uses both hands either side of the lower pole of the uterus, fingers together, using finger pads, not tips. May need to encourage breathing exercises or bend knees slightly. Alternative Pawlik's grip uses one hand only to grasp presenting part (PP) – painful and not recommended. Woman encouraged to feel PP for herself

Rationale   To confirm presentation and engagement. Can be uncomfortable and cause woman to 'guard' her abdomen. To involve woman in her care

Findings   Head feels hard and smooth, neck distinguishable. Buttocks broad and no neck felt. If fingers when placed either side of head can get round top and point inwards = not engaged. If fingers point outward around base of head, likely to be engaged

---

contractions (non-stress test) is usually performed, often in an antenatal day unit (Andrews 2002). However, there is wide variation in midwives and obstetricians' responses to women reporting reduced fetal movements and further evidence is required in this area to inform appropriate management (Heazell et al 2008).

Fetal heart rate

It is not recommended by NICE (2008) to routinely listen to the fetal heart though a woman may find it comforting and may ask for a midwife to do so. The fetal heart can usually be detected using a Doppler, as soon as the

Activity

Imagine what advice you would give a woman who had not felt fetal movements by 20 weeks of pregnancy.

Think about what you would say to a woman who states that her baby does not seem to be moving as much as usual.

uterus is palpable above the symphysis pubis. It is often not possible to hear the fetal heart clearly through a Pinard's stethoscope (pinards) before 28 weeks' gestation. Wickham (2002) provides a useful summary of the 'tips and tricks' used by midwives when listening to the fetal heart through pinards.

Having identified the position of the fetal back during palpation, the midwife uses pinards (depending on gestation) to locate the fetal heart (in between the fetal shoulders). Clear location of the fetal heart also informs the identification of fetal position and presentation. It is essential that the midwife develops and maintains this clinical skill to avoid difficulty in the event of Doppler battery failure. It also enables the midwife to determine the best place to position the Doppler transducer, thus avoiding unnecessary noise distortion. The midwife can then use a Doppler so that the woman and her companion(s) can hear the fetal heart beat. The maternal pulse should also be identified to confirm that the heart rate detected abdominally is that of the fetus. It should be auscultated for a full minute and the number of

beats per minute (bpm) recorded in the woman's antenatal records. If the fetus becomes active during this time, acceleration of the fetal heart should be noted.

The fetal heart rate (FHR) varies according to gestational age. The mean FHR at 25 weeks' gestation is 150 bpm reducing to approximately 142 bpm at term (Park et al 2001). A reassuring fetal heart rate is between 110 and 160 bpm (NICE 2007). Any deviation from this range or irregularity detected requires referral to an obstetrician (NMC 2004).

Reflection on trigger scenario

Look back at the scenario:

Joanna is now 36 weeks into her pregnancy and feeling well but tired. The baby seems to be most active at night when she is trying to sleep – she doesn't seem to notice the movements during the day. Jo has developed some stretch marks at the top of her legs and is hoping they will not appear on her tummy as she likes wearing low-waisted jeans. Her partner has not yet heard the baby's heartbeat and is hoping to take time off work to go with Jo for her next antenatal appointment.

Now that you are familiar with monitoring fetal wellbeing you should have insight into how the scenario relates to the evidence about this. The jigsaw model will now be used to explore the trigger scenario in more depth.

Effective communication

During antenatal care it is important for a midwife to use communication skills appropriately. She will need to use her skills to find out information from Joanna in order to establish the wellbeing of Joanna and her baby. Questions that arise from the scenario might include: Has Joanna met her midwife before? What questions may the midwife ask her to find out what has been taking place? What clues may the midwife look for to establish Jo's feelings about the wellbeing of her baby? Where will the midwife record information?

Woman-centred care

This involves a sensitive, individualized approach to care and considering the woman's needs from her perspective. In Jo's situation the midwife will consider her thoughts and needs at this time. Questions that arise from the scenario might include: What is concerning Jo most about the wellbeing of herself or her baby? How might the concerns about her stretch marks be addressed? How will her partner be included more in this pregnancy?

Using best evidence

In this scenario the midwife needs to consider the best evidence available to ensure fetal wellbeing is monitored effectively. Questions that arise from the scenario might include: Is there any evidence from Jo that the baby is not moving appropriately? Are there any physical factors that may influence the growth of the baby? What do the stretch marks signify? What is the evidence surrounding their prevention? Which evidence supports the clinical practice of the midwife?

Professional and legal issues

Midwives should always practise within the framework of their profession and the law. In this scenario questions that need to be addressed to ensure that the woman's care fulfils statutory obligations include: Has the midwife been appropriately trained to give antenatal care? Is she practising according to the rules of practice and code of professional conduct? Are there any local, national or international guidelines relating to Jo's care? What action should the midwife take if she detects an abnormality? How would she document her care?

Team working

Though community based midwives often work alone they are also based within a primary health environment that involves other health professionals. It is important that they communicate with each other: each may have a particular insight into Joanna's health status. Questions that need to be addressed in this scenario are: Are there any indications that Jo and her baby need to be referred to another professional? If so, who will this be? Where will the midwife record information for other health professionals? How will the midwife make contact with other health professionals if required?

Clinical dexterity

In this scenario the midwife will require skill and experience to palpate Jo's abdomen, without causing undue distress or harm, and to auscultate the fetal heart, if required. Questions that could arise are: Has the midwife received appropriate training in the skills required? Where will this examination be carried out? How will she ensure Jo retains her dignity? What will she use to hear the fetal heart? How will she estimate fetal growth? How will she maintain her skills and pass them on to others?

Models of care

There are currently a number of models of antenatal care practised by midwives in the UK. Monitoring the wellbeing of the fetus may be more ideally carried out by the same person each time, particularly in relation to monitoring fetal growth. In this situation, questions that could be raised are: Has this midwife met Jo before and so is able to make judgment on changes in the growth? Would continuity of care be beneficial in this situation? Is home-based care more beneficial in this situation? Are there other professional groups involved in Jo's care who would need informing?

Safe environment

All midwifery care should be carried out in a safe environment, for the woman, her family members and also for the midwife. Questions that could be asked about this scenario are: Are Jo and her midwife safe within the environment of care? Is any of the equipment to be used likely to put her or her baby in danger? Are there any risks to the midwife with the position in which Jo will need to be examined? How could this be altered to prevent this risk?

Promotes health

Antenatal care provides many opportunities for midwives to promote the wellbeing of the woman, her baby and her family. In this scenario questions that could be asked to ensure that the woman's care promotes physical and emotional health include: Are there any lifestyle issues that may be affecting Jo or the baby's health? How will the midwife find this out? What suggestions may she make to help? What suggestions may she make regarding her anxieties? How may the midwife include the partner more in antenatal care?

Further scenarios

The following scenarios enable you to consider how specific situations influence the care the midwife provides. Use the jigsaw model to explore the issues raised in the scenario.

Scenario 1

Lisa is 39 weeks pregnant. Her husband comes home from work and says lightheartedly, 'How's nipper doing today?'. Lisa sits down and suddenly realizes that she has not noticed the baby move today.

Practice point

Further questions specific to Scenario 1 include:

1. When did Lisa last see her midwife?
2. Had there been any cause for concern at the last antenatal appointment?
3. Why might Lisa not have noticed the baby move today?
4. What should she do now?
5. What advice would you give her if you were her community midwife?

Scenario 2

Janice is 34 weeks pregnant. Although she has been trying really hard not to put too much weight on this time, she is already classified as 'obese'. Last time she went to clinic for a routine antenatal appointment the midwife referred her to the hospital for an ultrasound scan.

Practice point

Further questions specific to Scenario 2 include:

1. Why did the midwife refer Janice for a scan?

2. What factors influence the growth of the fetus?
3. In what circumstances can it be difficult to estimate gestational age through symphysis pubis measurement?
4. What other parameters are used to assess fetal wellbeing during routine care?
5. How should Janice's remaining care be managed?

Conclusion

Monitoring fetal wellbeing in the community setting requires the use of the midwife's skill in the clinical art of abdominal palpation. During this systematic examination the midwife not only uses her hands to confirm that the fetus is growing and active but uses her interpersonal skills to enable the woman to take an active part in monitoring her baby's health.

Resources

External cephalic version: National Childbirth Trust. http://www.nct.org.uk/info-centre/a-to-z/view/203.

Information regarding customised fetal growth charts. http://www.perinatal.nhs.uk/growth/index_growth.htm.

National Institute for Health and Clinical Excellence. http://www.nice.org.uk/.

Optimum fetal positioning: Home birth website. http://www.homebirth.org.uk/ofp.htm.

Royal College of Obstetricians and Gynaecologists. http://www.rcog.org.uk/.

References

Andrews S: The antenatal CTG, *The Practising Midwife* 5(9):18–20, 2002.

Berbey R, Manduley A, Gracia VG: Counting fetal movements as a universal test for fetal wellbeing, *International Journal of Gynecology and Obstetrics* 74(3):293–295, 2001.

Berghella V: Prevention of recurrent fetal growth restriction, *Obstetrics and Gynecology* 110(4):904–912, 2007.

Engstrom JL, Ostrenga KG, Plass RV, et al: The effect of maternal bladder volume on fundal height measurements, *British Journal of Obstetrics and Gynaecology* 96(8):987–991, 1989.

Engstrom JL, Sittler CP: Fundal height measurement. Part 1 – techniques for measuring fundal height, *Journal of Nurse Midwifery* 38(1):5–16, 1993.

Engstrom JL, McFarlin B, Sittler CP: Fundal height measurement. Part 2 – intra- and interexaminer reliability of three measurement techniques, *Journal of Nurse Midwifery* 38(1):17–22, 1993a.

Engstrom JL, Piscioneri L, Low LK, et al: Fundal height measurement. Part 3 – the effect of maternal position on fundal height measurements, *Journal of Nurse Midwifery* 38(1):23–27, 1993b.

Enkin M, Keirse MJNC, Neilson J, et al: *A guide to effective care in pregnancy and childbirth*, ed 3, Oxford, 2000, Oxford University Press.

Gardosi J, Francis A: Controlled trial of fundal height measurement plotted on customised antenatal growth charts, *British Journal of Obstetrics and Gynaecology* 106:309–317, 1999.

Heazell A, Green M, Wright C, et al: Midwives and obstetrician knowledge and management of women presenting with decreased fetal movements, *Acta Obstetrica et Gynecologica Scandinavica* 87(3):331–339, 2008.

James D: Assessing fetal health, *Current Obstetrics and Gynaecology* 12(5):243–249, 2002.

Mangesi L, Hofmeyr GJ: Fetal movement counting for assessment of fetal wellbeing, Accessed 30/4/08. *Cochrane Database of Systematic Reviews* 1(CD004909), 2007.

McGeown P: Detecting fetal growth abnormalities, *MIDIRS Midwifery Digest* 11(2):190–193, 2001.

National Institute for Health and Clinical Excellence (NICE): *Intrapartum care. Care of healthy women and their babies during childbirth. NICE Clinical Guideline 55*, London, 2007, NICE.

National Institute for Health and Clinical Excellence (NICE): *Antenatal care: routine care for the healthy pregnant woman*, 2008. Online. Available http://www.nice.org.uk/guidance/index.jsp?action= byID&o=11947. April 4, 2008.

Neilson J: Symphysis – fundal height measurement in pregnancy (Cochrane Review) No: CD000944. Accesssed 30/4/09. In *The Cochrane Library*, Oxford, 1998, Update Software.

Nursing and Midwifery Council (NMC): *Midwives rules and standards*, London, 2004, NMC.

Nursing and Midwifery Council (NMC): *Standards for pre-registration midwifery education*, London, 2009, NMC.

Park MI, Hwang JH, Cha KJ, et al: Computerized analysis of fetal heart rate parameters by gestational age, *International Journal of Gynecology & Obstetrics* 74(2):157–164, 2001.

Perinatal Institute: Assessment of fetal growth using customised growth charts: NICE antenatal care guidelines vs Best practice, 2008. Online. Available http://www.perinatal.nhs.uk/nice/index.htm. April 30, 2008.

Statham H, Green J, Kafetsios K: Who worries that something might be wrong with the baby? A prospective study of 1072 pregnant women, *Birth* 24(4):223–233, 1997.

Wickham S: Pinard wisdom. Tips and tricks from midwives (Part 1), *The Practising Midwife* 5(9):21, 2002.

Young GL, Jewell D: Creams for preventing stretch marks in pregnancy, *Cochrane Database of Systematic Reviews 1996* 2(CD000066), 1996.

Zhang X, Platt RW, Cnattingius S, et al: The use of customised versus population-based birth weight standards in predicting perinatal mortality, *British Journal of Obstetrics and Gynecology* 114(4):474–477, 2007.

Chapter 10

Antenatal care: preparing for the birth

Trigger scenario

Joanna is now 36 weeks into her pregnancy. She is worried about how her partner, Louis, will support her during labour. Although he has been to a couple of classes, there seems to be only one man who says anything and he has been through the process with another partner. Joanna feels that it is really important to her that Louis takes an active role during the labour. However, she worries that he may be overwhelmed and not feel comfortable with the situation.

Introduction

This chapter explores the preparations made by women and their partners as they approach the birth of their baby. Issues including antenatal expectations and preparation for childbirth classes will be considered. The use of birth plans as a tool to enable women and their birthing partners to discuss and clarify hopes and fears about the labour and birth will also be outlined.

Antenatal expectations

Many women will approach birth with a complex set of hopes and concerns. These will reflect many influences including their previous experiences, the stories they have been told (Weston 2001) and their personality (Saisto et al 2001a). In some instances, the anticipation of the unknown generates fear of childbirth (Wijma et al 1998) as highlighted in Chapter 6. The evidence is not clear regarding the most appropriate intervention to help women overcome this fear. In a study by Ryding et al (2003) it was found that women who had consulted specially trained midwives because of fear of childbirth during pregnancy reported a more frightening experience of birth than women in the comparison group. Saisto et al (2001b) randomly allocated women who had presented with fear of vaginal birth to either a combination of cognitive therapy and written information (intensive therapy) or to information only (conventional therapy). They found that women in the intensive therapy group had shorter labours and that birth-related anxiety was reduced. There was no difference, however, between the two groups in the incidence of postnatal depression.

How women anticipate birth has significant sequelae for their experiences. In a large prospective study exploring women's expectations and experiences of childbirth (Green et al 2003) it was reported that women in 2000 were significantly more worried antenatally about the thought of pain in labour, than women in 1987. This increase was particularly marked for primigravid women with 26% choosing the option 'very worried' compared with only 9% in 1987. Women in 2000 were also significantly more likely to accept obstetric intervention than their counterparts in 1987 (Green & Baston 2007). Midwives need to help women regain their faith in their ability to birth their babies without assistance. Further research is required to explore the most appropriate ways to enhance women's confidence and to facilitate and promote unassisted birth.

Preparation for birth classes

Women who have high expectations have better psychological outcomes than women who have low expectations (Slade et al 1993, Green et al 1998).

Women should be encouraged to develop confidence in their abilities to cope with the challenge of labour, and this should be one of the aims of preparation for childbirth classes. The provision of information about the choices available, such as pain relief, will enable women to be actively involved in decisions about their care. Involvement in decision-making is an important contributor to a positive birth experience, enhancing a woman's sense of control of the situation (Gibbens & Thomson 2001).

In a national survey of women's experience of maternity care conducted by the National Perinatology Epidemiology Unit (NPEU) (Redshaw et al 2006), 89% of first time mothers who responded said that they had been offered antenatal classes as part of their NHS care compared with 59% of women who had already had a baby. However, not all pregnant women who are offered classes take up the invitation; 33% of primigravid women and 80% of multgravid women did not attend. This may be for a range of reasons, including classes being full, not being held at convenient times or places, or not perceived as useful. Further subgroup analysis revealed that black and minority ethnic women were less likely to be offered classes, less likely to attend and less likely to attend with their partner than white women born in the United Kingdom.

The timing of local, community-based daytime classes may preclude many birth partners from attending classes with their pregnant partners. Provision should therefore be made in the evening or at weekends for those who want to attend. However, attendance at classes is not always reflected in a more positive experience of birth for fathers. In a study that aimed to explore if fathers' attendance at childbirth preparation classes influenced their experience of the birth (Greenhalgh et al 2000), it was reported that, for some fathers, attendance at classes was linked with a less positive appraisal of the childbirth experience. However, where men have been prepared as 'productive' participants in the labour process their involvement can have a positive impact on their partner's birth experience (Diemer 1997). It is important that all birth partners are involved and acknowledged for the support they provide. There is a need to provide childbirth preparation for men based on their expectations and individual perspective (Hallgren et al 1999). A report by the Fatherhood Institute (2008) highlights the lack of provision for the preparation of men for their role during childbirth. It calls for 'Relevant and securely funded NHS antenatal education that is appropriate to the needs of modern families and inclusive of fathers' (p. 8).

Activity

Find out what preparation for childbirth classes are available in your area. Find out what gestation they start at, who runs them and how many classes there are in a course.

Find out about Grantly Dick-Read. Who was he and what was his philosophy? What was his book called and what was the physiological basis for his ideas?

Depending on local provision, women should be encouraged to attend classes that best meet their individual needs. Classes for women who have already had a baby, for women expecting a multiple birth or for teenagers, are some examples of classes that cater for women's specific needs rather than the 'one class fits all' approach. The National Institute for Health and Clinical Excellence advises that women should be offered participant-led antenatal classes and breastfeeding workshops (NICE 2008).

Non-NHS classes

The provision of non-NHS classes has grown significantly. This may be in response to lack of availability but also to the desire to have a more personal experience, rather than attend a large anonymous group at the hospital. In the NPEU survey (Redshaw et al 2006) it was reported that 6% of women paid for their antenatal classes. Private classes range from a luxury weekend away with like-minded couples to yoga and hypnobirthing coaching.

Physical preparation

Women can also make physical preparations for the birth. These may include attending activities designed especially for pregnant women, such as aquanatal and relaxation sessions. Preparations can also be made for an active labour by becoming familiar with and practising strategies to cope with contractions using non-pharmacological means. Women should be informed of the potential benefits of the strategies available, to ensure they have realistic expectations of their effectiveness (Spiby et al 2003). Fletcher (2003) outlines the National Childbirth Trust's campaign 'Don't take it lying down', designed to encourage women to remain upright and mobile in labour. She argues that midwives can influence the positions that women adopt during labour by the way they either react to or facilitate the creation of an environment conducive to active birth. Women can be made to feel that the delivery room is theirs to adapt to their own needs or, alternatively, be made to feel that their requests or suggestions are too difficult to accommodate. The NPEU survey (Redshaw et al 2006) reported that 88.5% of all women who had a vaginal birth, did so on a bed, 6.1% on the floor and 4% in water. Multiparous women were more likely to give birth on the bed (15%) compared with primiparous women (7%).

Student midwives can play a significant role in helping women feel that their hopes and aspirations for the birth will be acknowledged and upheld wherever possible. The fresh knowledge and enthusiasm that the student midwife brings to clinical practice can contribute to the introduction of alternative ways of working, under the close supervision of experienced midwives.

Activity

Undertake an internet search for 'birth plans'. Look at some of the examples.

Decide whether the requests appear appropriate.

Imagine that you were approaching the birth of your first child. Think about what you would consider including in a birth plan and how you would justify your choices?

Birth plans

Government policy advocates that women should be able to make choices about their place of birth and use of pain relief, and that they should be given sufficient information in an accessible way, to help them make informed decisions (Department of Health 2007). Preparation for childbirth classes can be a valuable resource for women when it comes to making choices about what happens to them during labour. However, not all women are able or want to attend. Some women formalize their decisions before labour by completing a birth plan. This is a written outline of a woman's wishes for her birth. It may cover issues such as what kind of pain relief she would prefer, whether or not she wants to have electronic fetal monitoring and what position she would like to give birth in.

The use of birth plans has escalated in recent years and forms part of the National Maternity Records. There are many other alternative versions and examples available to women who have access to the internet. Some take the form of written lists created by the woman indicating the conditions in which certain interventions will be acceptable and when they will not. Others include a general philosophy of parents' hopes and aspirations for the circumstances in which their baby will be born. Many units use their own particular format to facilitate the birth planning process, often including a tick-box list with some room for specific comments. Although they have the advantage of providing structure to a discussion, they may not reflect the interests of the woman or encourage her to think about what she really wants (Nolan 2001). Kaufman (2008) describes how birth plans can take different forms, such as mind maps and decision trees, to help the woman explore how she feels about the birth. The popularity of birth plans has fluctuated, and they are sometimes seen as a hindrance by professionals rather than a tool to enhance woman-centred care. Simkin (2007) argues that birth plans do have a place in contemporary maternity care; that women still want to be heard and there are practitioners who use them respectfully to enhance the woman's sense of control.

Completion of a birth plan provides a useful opportunity for the woman to discuss the available options for the management of her care (Kaufman 2008), whether at home or in hospital. Their use may help to enhance communication between all members of the multi-professional team (Enkin

et al 2000). Some Trusts have specific policies and targets in relation to the completion of this aspect of the maternity notes, whereas other units do not formally dedicate either time or documentation to this activity. Where the birth plan forms part of routine care, this provides dedicated time for the midwife and woman to spend time together where the focus of the interaction is not abdominal palpation or blood pressure measurement. However, in reality, it may be combined with an antenatal examination.

In ideal circumstances, the midwife would visit the woman at home to discuss the birth plan. One of the main advantages of undertaking this activity in the woman's home is that she is more likely to feel relaxed and able to ask questions in an environment in which she has control. Meeting the woman on her own ground also provides the midwife with much valuable information about the circumstances in which the woman lives and in which she will care for her new baby.

Implementing birth plans

A study based on the responses of 101 primiparous women (Whitford & Hillan 1998) found that 90% of respondents had completed a birth plan. However, most women (60%) experienced some deviation from the plan, and 32% felt that the midwife did not read their plans. In a large prospective study undertaken by Green et al (1998) fewer than half of those who used birth plans felt that they had been helpful and 12% stated that their birth plans had been totally ignored by staff. Those women who were positive about the use of birth plans believed that they would be a useful tool to facilitate communication with staff, whereas those who were negative about their use felt that they might obstruct such interaction. Indeed, 25% of these women stated that a disadvantage of using a birth plan was that it might 'get you labelled as a trouble-maker' (Green et al 1998:287).

Nolan (2001) makes the point that women are unlikely to make unrealistic, inflexible requests if they have had the opportunity to discuss the birth plan with a midwife. Misconceptions or requests that would be difficult to meet can be discussed before the labour begins. A mutually agreed resolution can usually be found, thus avoiding conflict and disappointment on the labour ward.

Midwives need to be very careful that they do not withhold information about the choices available to women because of stereotypes that they hold. Kirkham et al (2002) found that midwives sometimes made judgments about the relevance or appropriateness of some kinds of information leaflets to particular groups of women. For example, one midwife stated that 'the young girls don't tend to be that interested' (p. 549), yet subsequent interviews with pregnant teenagers revealed that they deeply valued the information they contained. Indeed, a study of the information needs of first-time pregnant women found no significant difference in the information needs of women of different ethnic, age or socio-economic groups (Singh et al 2002). Similarly, Green et al (1990) reported that more educated women were no more committed to the idea of a drug-free birth than other women.

The partner's role

Completion of a birth plan is also an opportunity to involve the partner in preparations for the birth. Beardshaw (2001) argues that there is a strong case for providing information to prospective fathers and assisting them with the development of skills that will enable them to provide effective support for their partners. A study by Chan & Paterson-Brown (2002), involving 86 fathers and 88 mothers, concluded that fathers underestimated how helpful they had been to their partners during labour. Their significant positive contribution to the birth experience when undertaking a supportive role should be emphasized.

A systematic review of caregiver support during labour (provided by either lay people or professionals) found that the continuous presence of a support person in labour reduced the likelihood of operative delivery and the need for analgesia (Hodnett et al 2007). When men take on the role of birth partner, however, they can often feel overawed, and have difficulty coping with their partner's pain (Kunjappy-Clifton 2008).

Activity

Think about how the midwife can encourage birth partners to actively support the labouring woman.

Consider what antenatal preparations they can make together to facilitate this process.

List 10 ways the partner can participate during the labour.

Place of birth

One of the many advantages of having a home birth is that both the woman and her partner are already familiar with their surroundings. Women who choose to birth their baby in hospital are often coming into an environment that feels strange to them. Wouldn't it be nice if, before we went on holiday, we had a clear idea of the equipment and resources that would be available during our stay? We are not suggesting that coming into hospital to have a baby is like going on holiday, but there are certain useful parallels that can be drawn. Of course, the woman will not be wishing she had packed her travel iron, but she may wish she had packed her favourite tapes or CDs if she finds a player in her room.

Some women have had an opportunity to look around the labour ward before the birth, accompanied by a midwife who is familiar with the set-up. Such a 'guided tour' might have been part of her local antenatal classes, where the group arranges to meet at the delivery suite at an agreed date and

time. Alternatively, some labour wards have a 'guided tour' perhaps once a week, when a midwife who works there takes women, including those who are not attending classes or who could not get to their own tour, around the area.

Such a tour should ideally include not only a walk around the layout but also explanations about the function of some of the equipment. It is useful, for example, if the woman is familiar with what a fetal monitor looks like just in case one is used during her labour. Women may have heard that theatre is nearby and easily accessible in the event of an emergency, but being shown the physical location may be reassuring. Some units provide 'virtual' tours (web or DVD) of their facilities. This enables the maternity unit to be 'seen' at any time of day, without disturbing the privacy of the resident women.

Having a look around the maternity unit will help women decide what they need to take with them into hospital to make their stay more comfortable. Each maternity unit will vary in terms of the facilities it provides. Where possible, the woman should be encouraged to wear her own clothes and retain her own individuality and identity. She will need to take in items of clothing for the baby and to prepare clothes that she wants the baby to come home from hospital in, ready to be brought in on the day they go home. The partner will also need to prepare a small bag including energy-packed snacks, a camera and a list of who to phone when the baby arrives.

Women in special circumstances

When it is expected that a baby is likely to be admitted to the special care baby unit (SCBU) or transitional care ward, then prospective parents are likely to benefit by becoming familiar with the surroundings and meeting a member of staff before the baby is born.

Activity

Think about the circumstances in which a woman might expect her baby to be cared for in a special care baby unit.

Consider how this environment differs from a transitional care facility.

When to call a midwife

Diagnosing the onset of labour can be difficult, particularly for women expecting their first baby. They may be worried about initiating an unecessary trip to the hospital or conversely, concerned that they might not get to the hospital on time. A review of the evidence on self-diagnosis of the onset of active labour (Lauzon & Hodnett 2007) concluded that there was insufficient evidence that giving women specific criteria was any better than general guidelines. Whether the woman is expecting a home or a hospital birth, she should be in no doubt about the circumstances in which she should seek professional advice.

Often the local hospital, usually the labour ward, provides a central role in coordinating the enquiries of women who think they might be in labour or experiencing other problems. Alternatively, some women have direct access to their own community midwife who can assess the situation and provide advice and information for women on her caseload.

The woman should be advised to speak to a midwife if she has:

- Bleeding or abnormal vaginal discharge
- Spontaneous rupture of membranes (SROM)
- Severe itching
- Severe headache, visual disturbance or epigastric pain
- Reduced/excessive fetal movements
- Regular, painful contractions, building in frequency, length and intensity.

The midwife should be contacted at the onset of contractions if the woman is booked for elective caesarean section, has a breech presentation, a pre-existing medical condition, a multiple pregnancy, a previous precipitate labour or is not at term.

Activity

Think about the facilities available in your unit for women and their partners.

If you were compiling a list of items that a woman might find useful in hospital, think about what it would include. Make a list of things she would need to bring in for her baby during the hospital stay.

Reflection on trigger scenario

Look back on the trigger scenario.

Joanna is now 36 weeks into her pregnancy. She is worried about how her partner, Louis, will support her during labour. Although he has been to a couple of classes, there seems to be only one man who says anything and he has been through the process with another partner. Joanna feels that it is really important to her that Louis takes an active role during the labour. However, she worries that he may be overwhelmed and not feel comfortable with the situation.

Now that you are familiar with issues around preparation for birth you should have insight into how the scenario relates to the evidence. The jigsaw model will now be used to explore the trigger scenario in more depth.

Effective communication

The midwife needs to communicate effectively with the pregnant woman and her birth partner when she prepares them for the impending birth. She has access to a range of resources to help her do this: one model is the birth plan. Questions that arise from the scenario might include: Has Joanna considered completing a birth plan? Has the midwife encouraged her to do this? Has Louis communicated his hopes and fears about the birth to Joanna? Has Joanna talked to Louis about how much she wants him to be involved in the birth? Does he know how important this is to Jo?

Woman-centred care

Attending antenatal classes is one way that prospective parents can get information to enable them to make informed decisions about their care. It also provides an opportunity to explore hopes and fears for birth with their peer group. Questions that arise from the scenario might include: Are the classes participant-led? Does everyone get the opportunity to voice their individual concerns and aspirations for the birth? How can antenatal classes be facilitated to ensure that they meet the needs of the group rather than the needs of the organization? Are there any opportunities for prospective fathers to get together as a group?

Using best evidence

A range of evidence informs all aspects of maternity care. Accessing appropriate and relevant information is also a challenge for women and their partners. Questions that arise from the scenario might include: What are the benefits of attending preparation for childbirth classes, for the woman and her partner? Is there evidence to support one model of parent education over another? What is the evidence to support Jo's aspirations for the active involvement of her partner during labour and birth?

Professional and legal issues

It is part of the midwife's professional role to 'provide a programme of parenthood preparation; (NMC 2004:37). The midwife can help facilitate a positive birth experience for Joanna and Louis, by actively taking her wishes into consideration.

Questions that arise from the scenario might include: What organizational factors might prevent the midwife from actioning Joanna's preferences for labour management? In what circumstances might the midwife need to abandon Joanna's plans for labour? What action should the midwife take if Joanna requested a form of care that the midwife perceives to be unsafe?

Team working

Preparing prospective parents for the birth is predominantly the remit of the midwife. However, there are other key professionals who make an important contribution to this preparation. For example, in some areas, the health visitor, infant feeding advisor, physiotherapist and maternity support worker have a role to play. Questions that arise from the scenario might include: How might the midwife help Joanna to involve Louis in preparing for the birth? Who might be the most appropriate person to listen to Louis's concerns about the birth?

Clinical dexterity

Midwives work in a range of clinical settings and across the childbirth continuum. They need to keep up-to-date with all aspects of current practice. Questions that arise from the scenario might include: How can community midwives, providing preparation for childbirth classes for women, keep up-to-date with current practice in hospital intrapartum care? What educational resources are available for use in antenatal classes? Are there any education programmes for midwives to help them develop their teaching skills?

Models of care

Preparation for childbirth classes should take account of the various choices that women make regarding the model of care most appropriate for them. Questions that arise from the scenario might include: How might the place of birth impact on Louis's confidence to support Joanna throughout her labour and birth? Is there an opportunity for Louis to become familiar with the birth environment? What model(s) of care would facilitate or hinder the development of trusting relationships between the midwife and her clients?

Safe environment

Sometimes partners feel 'like a spare part' during their partner's labour, lacking the confidence to be an active carer in front of professionals. They need to feel safe to get involved and participate in the process of birth. Questions that arise from the scenario might include: What steps can the midwife take to involve Louis in Joanna's care, before she comes into hospital? How can he be supported to continue to support Joanna when she comes into hospital? What aspects of the physical labour ward environment can be changed to facilitate the active involvement of birth partners?

Promotes health

Women vary in the degree of support they want or expect from their partner. For some, the active support of their partner is felt to be an integral part of the birth experience. Joanna's emotional health is at risk if she has unrealistic expectations of the support that Louis can provide during labour. Questions that arise from the scenario might include: How can Joanna and Louis gain a mutual understanding of each other's expectations for the birth? How can the midwife facilitate this?

Further scenarios

The following scenarios enable you to consider how specific situations influence the care the midwife provides. Use the jigsaw model to explore the issues raised in the scenario.

Scenario 1

Julie is expecting her second baby. Although her first child is only 3 years old, he was born by elective caesarean and Julie feels very nervous about the prospect of labour. She has never accessed antenatal classes and is now fearful that she will not be able to cope with her contractions.

Practice point

Further questions specific to Scenario 1 include:

1. Why did Julie have an elective caesarean with her first baby?

2. Was Julie offered antenatal classes in her first pregnancy?
3. If so, why did she not access them?
4. Was Julie offered antenatal classes this time around?
5. How can Julie be prepared to go into labour with confidence?
6. Has she got a birth partner and if so, what preparation have they had?

Scenario 2

Elizabeth is a school teacher and she has just arrived on the labour ward with a history of regular contractions for the last 2 hours. After the last contraction, the midwife asks her what she wants for her pain. Elizabeth replies that she has been to National Childbirth Trust (NCT) classes and would like to avoid using any pharmacological pain relief, if at all possible.

Practice point

Further questions specific to Scenario 2 include:

1. What pre-conceived ideas do you have about Elizabeth's level of education and her aspirations for birth?
2. What pre-conceived ideas do you have about NCT antenatal classes?
3. What evidence do you have on which to base your assumptions?
4. What actions can you take to ensure that your information is reliable?
5. What action can you take to show respect for Elizabeth's hopes for a drug-free labour?

Conclusion

The unpredictability of the onset and course of labour makes it a difficult event to plan and prepare for. With so many different expectations and experiences to consider, the midwife must assess each woman's situation in order to help her prepare for the birth. The student midwife has a valuable role to play in helping a woman feel that her specific situation is understood and her hopes respected.

Resources

Campaign for normal birth: http://www.rcmnormalbirth.org.uk/.

Fatherhood Institute's research summary: maternal and infant health in the perinatal period: the father's role. http://www.fatherhoodinstitute.org/uploads/publications/356.pdf.

Home birth plans: http://www.homebirth.org.uk/plan.htm.

La Leche League (LLL): http://www.laleche.org.uk/.

The National Childbirth Trust (NCT): http://www.nctpregnancyandbabycare.com/home.

NHS Direct. Making choices during pregnancy. http://www.nhs.uk/planners/pregnancycareplanner/Pages/PregnancyHome.aspx.

References

Beardshaw T: Supporting the role of fathers around the time of birth, *MIDIRS Midwifery Digest* 11(4):476–479, 2001.

Chan K, Paterson-Brown S: How do fathers feel after accompanying their partners in labour and delivery? *Journal of Obstetrics and Gynaecology* 22(1): 11–15, 2002.

Department of Health: *Maternity matters: choice, access and continuity of care in a safe service*, London, 2007, Department of Health.

Diemer G: Expectant fathers: influence of perinatal education on coping, stress, and spousal relations, *Research in Nursing and Health* 20:281–293, 1997.

Enkin M, Keirse M, Neilson J, et al: *A guide to effective care in pregnancy and childbirth*, ed 3, Oxford, 2000, Oxford University Press.

Fatherhood Institute: The dad deficit: the missing piece of the maternity jigsaw, 2008. Online. Available http://www.fatherhoodinstitute.org/index.php?id=2&cID=735. April 29, 2008.

Fletcher G: Don't take it lying down! *The Practising Midwife* 6(2):14–15, 2003.

Gibbens J, Thomson A: Women's expectations and experiences of childbirth, *Midwifery* 17(4):302–313, 2001.

Green J, Kitzinger J, Coupland V: Stereotypes of childbearing women: a look at some evidence, *Midwifery* 6:125–132, 1990.

Green J, Coupland V, Kitzinger J: *Great expectations. A prospective study of women's expectations and experiences of childbirth*, Hale, 1998, Books for Midwives Press.

Green J, Baston H, Easton S, et al: *Greater expectations? Inter-relationships between expectations and experiences of decision making, continuity, choice and control in labour, and psychological outcomes. Summary report*, Leeds, 2003, University of Leeds, Mother & Infant Research Unit.

Green JM, Baston HA: Have women become more willing to accept obstetric interventions and does this relate to mode of birth? Data from a prospective study, *Birth* 34(1): 6–13, 2007.

Greenhalgh R, Slade P, Spiby H: Fathers' coping style, antenatal preparation, and experiences of labor and the postpartum, *Birth* 27(3): 177–184, 2000.

Hallgren A, Kihlgren M, Forslin L, et al: Swedish fathers' involvement in and experiences of childbirth preparation and childbirth, *Midwifery* 15(1):6–15, 1999.

Hodnett ED, Gates S, Hofmeyr GJ, et al: Continuous support for women during childbirth, *Cochrane Database of Systematic Reviews* 2(CD003766), 2007.

Kaufman T: Evolution of the birth plan, *MIDIRS Midwifery Digest* 18(1):67–70, 2008.

Kirkham M, Stapleton H, Curtis P, et al: Stereotyping as a professional defence mechanism, *British Journal of Midwifery* 10(9):549–552, 2002.

Kunjappy-Clifton A: And father came too. A study exploring the role of first time fathers during the birth process and to explore the meaning of the experience for these men. Part 2, *MIDIRS Midwifery Digest* 18(1):57–66, 2008.

Lauzon L, Hodnett E: Antenatal education for self-diagnosis of the onset of active labour at term, *Cochrane Database of Systematic Reviews*(CD000935), 2007.

National Institute of Health and Clinical Excellence (NICE): *Antenatal care: routine care for the healthy pregnant woman. Clinical guideline 62*, London, 2008, National Collaborating Centre for Women's and Children's Health.

Nolan M: Birth plans. A relic of the past or still a useful tool? *The Practising Midwife* 4(5):38–39, 2001.

Nursing and Midwifery Council (NMC): *Midwives rules and standards*, London, 2004, NMC.

Redshaw M, Rowe R, Hockley C, et al: *Recorded delivery: a national survey of women's experience of maternity care*, Oxford, 2006, National Perinatal Epidemiology Unit.

Ryding EL, Persson A, Onell C, et al: An evaluation of midwives' counseling of pregnant women in fear of childbirth, *Acta Obstetrica et Gynecologica Scandinavica* 82: 10–17, 2003.

Saisto T, Salmela-Aro K, Nurmi J-E, et al: Psychosocial characteristics of women and their partners fearing vaginal childbirth, *British Journal of Obstetrics and Gynaecology* 108(5): 492–498, 2001a.

Saisto T, Salmela-Aro K, Nurmi J-E, et al: A randomised controlled trial of intervention in fear of childbirth, *Obstetrics and Gynaecology* 98(5Pt1):820–826, 2001b.

Simkin P: Birth plans: after 25 years, women still want to be heard, *Birth* 34(1):49–51, 2007.

Singh D, Newburn M, Smith N, et al: The information needs of first-time pregnant mothers, *British Journal of Midwifery* 10(1):54–58, 2002.

Slade P, MacPherson S, Hume A, et al: Expectations, experiences and satisfaction with labour, *British Journal of Clinical Psychology* 32:469–483, 1993.

Spiby H, Slade P, Escott D, et al: Selected coping strategies in labour: an investigation of women's experiences, *Birth* 30(3):189–194, 2003.

Weston R: The influence of birth stories from friends and family members on primigravid women, *MIDIRS Midwifery Digest* 11(4):495–500, 2001.

Whitford H, Hillan E: Women's perceptions of birth plans, *Midwifery* 14(4):248–253, 1998.

Wijma K, Wijma B, Zar M: Psychometric aspects of the W-DEQ; a new questionnaire for the measurement of fear of childbirth, *Journal of Psychosomatic Obstetrics and Gynaecology* 19:84–97, 1998.

A

abdominal inspection
    scars 125
    shape 124–5
    size 126
    skin 125–6
abdominal palpation 124, 125, 126, 129
    fundal 128–9
    gestational age 126–8
    lateral 128–9
    pelvic 128–9
aching legs 50
aims of antenatal care 10
alcohol 28, 44–5
antenatal care
    aims of 10
    NICE guidelines 58–9, 60–1
    planning 32
    preparation for birth 136–47
antenatal care models 8–17
    caseload midwifery 15
    consultant care 16
    group practice 15
    independent midwifery practice 15–16
    integrated care 14
    midwife-led care 13
    shared care 13
    Sure Start 15
    team midwifery 14
antenatal check 58–62
    emotional wellbeing 61–2
    fetal wellbeing 122–33
    record keeping 59
    safety 59, 61
    social activity 62

antenatal classes 137–8
    non-NHS 138
antenatal depression 78
antenatal screening 24, 106–19
    definition of 106–7
    diagnostic tests 114–16
    Down's syndrome 108–13
    false positive/negative 107–8
    haemoglobinopathies 113–14
    structural abnormalities 114
anti-D 96–7

B

backache 58
best evidence 2–3
birth plans 139–41
    implementation 140–1
Birth Under Midwifery Practice Scheme (BUMPS) 15
blood group 94–7
blood pressure measurement 64
blood tests 64, 90–102
    blood group and rhesus factor 94–7
    full blood count 92–4
    hepatitis B virus 99
    human immunodeficiency virus 98
    red cell antibodies 97
    rubella antibodies 97–8
    syphilis 98
body image 74–5
body mass index 31, 41
booking history 20–35
    antenatal care planning 32
    antenatal screening 24
    communication 22–3
    developing relationships 21–3
    information 22